T0127862

Measuring Sleep

Editor

ERNA SIF ARNARDOTTIR

SLEEP MEDICINE CLINICS

www.sleep.theclinics.com

December 2021 • Volume 16 • Number 4

ELSEVIER

1600 John F. Kennedy Boulevard • Suite 1800 • Philadelphia, Pennsylvania, 19103-2899

http://www.theclinics.com

SLEEP MEDICINE CLINICS Volume 16, Number 4
December 2021, ISSN 1556-407X, ISBN-13: 978-0-323-89760-0

Editor: Joanna Collett
Developmental Editor: Axell Ivan Jade M. Purificacion

Sleep Medicine Clinics (ISSN 1556-407X) is published quarterly by Elsevier Inc., 360 Park Avenue South, New York, NY 10010-1710. Months of issue are March, June, September and December. Business and Editorial Offices: 1600 John F. Kennedy Blvd., Ste. 1800, Philadelphia, PA 19103-2899. Customer Service Office: 3251 Riverport Lane, Maryland Heights, MO 63043. Periodicals postage paid at New York, NY and additional mailing offices. Subscription prices are $225.00 per year (US individuals), $100.00 (US and Canadian students), $625.00 (US institutions), $272.00 (Canadian individuals), $252.00 (international individuals) $135.00 (International students), $656.00 (Canadian and International institutions). Foreign air speed delivery is included in all *Clinics* subscription prices. All prices are subject to change without notice. **POSTMASTER:** Send change of address to *Sleep Medicine Clinics*, Elsevier Health Sciences Division, Subscription Customer Service, 3251 Riverport Lane, Maryland Heights, MO 63043. Customer Service: **Tel: 1-800-654-2452 (U.S. and Canada); 314-447-8871 (outside U.S. and Canada). Fax: 314-447-8029. E-mail: journalscustomerservice-usa@elsevier.com (for print support); journalsonline-support-usa@elsevier.com (for online support)**.

Reprints. For copies of 100 or more of articles in this publication, please contact the Commercial Reprints Department, Elsevier Inc., 360 Park Avenue South, New York, NY 10010-1710. Tel.: 212-633-3874; Fax: 212-633-3820; E-mail: reprints@elsevier.com.

Sleep Medicine Clinics is covered in *MEDLINE/PubMed (Index Medicus)*.

SLEEP MEDICINE CLINICS

SERIES OF RELATED INTEREST

Neurologic Clinics
Available at: https://www.neurologic.theclinics.com/

THE CLINICS ARE AVAILABLE ONLINE!
Access your subscription at:
www.theclinics.com

Contributors

CONSULTING EDITOR

TEOFILO LEE-CHIONG Jr, MD
Professor of Medicine, National Jewish Health,
University of Colorado Denver, Denver,
Colorado; Chief Medical Liaison, Philips
Respironics, Pennsylvania

ANA C. KRIEGER, MD
Chief, Division of Sleep Neurology Medical
Director, Weill Cornell Center for Sleep
Medicine, Professor of Clinical Medicine,
Professor of Medicine in Neurology and
Genetic Medicine, New York, USA

EDITOR

ERNA SIF ARNARDOTTIR, PhD
Assistant Professor and Director, Reykjavik
University Sleep Institute, School of
Technology, Reykjavik University, Internal
Medicine Services, Landspitali–The National
University Hospital of Iceland, Reykjavik,
Iceland

AUTHORS

BIRTA SÓLEY ÁRNADÓTTIR, BSc
Research Assistant, Department of
Psychology, Reykjavik University Sleep
Institute, School of Technology, Reykjavik
University, Reykjavik, Iceland

ERNA SIF ARNARDOTTIR, PhD
Assistant Professor and Director, Reykjavik
University Sleep Institute, School of
Technology, Reykjavik University, Internal
Medicine Services, Landspitali-The National
University Hospital of Iceland, Reykjavik,
Iceland

SÉBASTIEN BAILLIEUL, MD, PhD
Department of Neurology, Bern University
Hospital (Inselspital) and University Bern,
Switzerland; Univ. Grenoble Alpes, Inserm,
U1300, CHU Grenoble Alpes, Service

Universitaire de Pneumologie Physiologie,
Grenoble, France

KELLY G. BARON, PhD
Division of Public Health, Department of Family
and Preventative Medicine, University of Utah,
Salt Lake City, Utah, USA

CLAUDIO L.A. BASSETTI, MD
Professor, Department of Neurology, Bern
University Hospital (Inselspital) and University
Bern, Switzerland; Department of Neurology,
University of Sechenow, Moscow, Russia

FRÉ A. BAUTERS, MD, PhD
Department of Respiratory Medicine, Ghent
University Hospital, Department of Internal
Medicine and Paediatrics, Faculty of Medicine
and Health Sciences, Ghent University, Gent,
Belgium

MARTIJN P.J. DEKKERS, MD, PhD
Department of Neurology, Bern University Hospital (Inselspital) and University Bern, Switzerland

CHRISTOPHER M. DEPNER, PhD
Department of Health and Kinesiology, University of Utah, Salt Lake City, Utah, USA

SARAH DIETZ-TERJUNG, MSc
Faculty of Sleep and Telemedicine, University Medicine Essen - Ruhrlandklinik, West German Lung Center, University Duisburg-Essen, Essen, Germany

AMIT KRISHNA DWIVEDI, PhD
Department of Applied Physics, University of Eastern Finland, Diagnostic Imaging Center, Kuopio University Hospital, Kuopio, Finland

DIMITRI FERRETTI, MSc
PhD Student, Reykjavik University Sleep Institute, School of Technology, Reykjavik University, Reykjavik, Iceland

LIVIA FREGOLENTE, MD
Department of Neurology, Bern University Hospital (Inselspital) and University Bern, Switzerland

ORIELLA GNARRA, MSc
Department of Neurology, Bern University Hospital (Inselspital) and University Bern, Switzerland; Sensory-Motor System Lab, IRIS, ETH Zurich, Switzerland

TANYA M. HALLIDAY, PhD
Department of Health and Kinesiology, University of Utah, Salt Lake City, Utah, USA

KATRIEN HERTEGONNE, MD, PhD
Department of Respiratory Medicine, Ghent University Hospital, Department of Internal Medicine and Paediatrics, Faculty of Medicine and Health Sciences, Ghent University, Gent, Belgium

KAMILLA RÚN JÓHANNSDÓTTIR, PhD
Associate Professor, Department of Psychology, Reykjavik University Sleep Institute, School of Technology, Reykjavik University, Reykjavik, Iceland

MARÍA KRISTÍN JÓNSDÓTTIR, PhD
Professor, Department of Psychology, Reykjavik University Sleep Institute, School of Technology, Reykjavik University, Landspitali University Hospital, Reykjavik, Iceland

JASMINE JENDOUBI, MSc
Department of Neurology, Bern University Hospital (Inselspital) and University Bern, Switzerland

SAMU KAINULAINEN, PhD
Department of Applied Physics, University of Eastern Finland, Diagnostic Imaging Center, Kuopio University Hospital, Kuopio, Finland

HENRI KORKALAINEN, PhD
Department of Applied Physics, University of Eastern Finland, Diagnostic Imaging Center, Kuopio University Hospital, Kuopio, Finland

TIMO LEPPÄNEN, PhD
Department of Applied Physics, University of Eastern Finland, Diagnostic Imaging Center, Kuopio University Hospital, Kuopio, Finland; School of Information Technology and Electrical Engineering, The University of Queensland, Brisbane, Australia

JACKY MALLETT, PhD
Department of Computer Science, Reykjavik University, Reykjavik, Iceland

WALTER T. McNICHOLAS, MD, FERS
Newman Professor, Department of Respiratory and Sleep Medicine, School of Medicine, University College Dublin, St. Vincent's Hospital Group, Dublin, Ireland

SAMI MYLLYMAA, PhD
Department of Applied Physics, University of Eastern Finland, Diagnostic Imaging Center, Kuopio University Hospital, Kuopio, Finland

SAMI NIKKONEN, PhD
Department of Applied Physics, University of Eastern Finland, Diagnostic Imaging Center, Kuopio University Hospital, Kuopio, Finland

THOMAS PENZEL, PhD
Interdisciplinary Sleep Medicine Center, Charité – Universitätsmedizin Berlin, Freie Universität Berlin, Humboldt-Universität zu Berlin, Berlin Institute of Health, Berlin, Germany; Department of Biology, Saratov State University, Saratov, Russia

DIRK PEVERNAGIE, MD, PhD
Department of Respiratory Medicine, Ghent University Hospital, Department of Internal Medicine and Paediatrics, Faculty of Medicine and Health Sciences, Ghent University, Gent, Belgium

FRIDA RÅNGTELL, PhD
Slumra of Sweden AB, Uppsala, Sweden

CHRISTOPH SCHÖBEL, MD, PhD
Faculty of Sleep and Telemedicine, University Medicine Essen - Ruhrlandklinik, West German Lung Center, University Duisburg-Essen, Essen, Germany

MARKUS H. SCHMIDT, MD, PhD
Department of Neurology, Bern University Hospital (Inselspital) and University Bern, Switzerland; Ohio Sleep Medicine Institute, Dublin, Ohio, USA

BARBARA GNIDOVEC STRAŽIŠAR, MD, PhD
Associate Professor, Pediatric Department, Centre for Pediatric Sleep Disorders, General Hospital Celje, Celje, Slovenia; College of Nursing in Celje, Celje, Slovenia; Medical Faculty, University of Maribor, Maribor, Slovenia

JUHA TÖYRÄS, PhD
Department of Applied Physics, University of Eastern Finland, Science Service Center, Kuopio University Hospital, Kuopio, Finland; School of Information Technology and Electrical Engineering, The University of Queensland, Brisbane, Australia

JENNY THEORELL-HAGLÖW, PhD
Department of Medical Sciences, Respiratory, Allergy and Sleep Research, Uppsala University, Uppsala, Sweden

SELENE Y. TOBIN, MS
Department of Health and Kinesiology, University of Utah, Salt Lake City, Utah, USA

MARTIN ULANDER, PhD
Department of Biomedical and Clinical Sciences, Faculty of Medicine, Linköping University, Department of Clinical Neurophysiology, Linköping University Hospital, Linköping, Sweden

ALBRECHT VORSTER, PhD
Department of Neurology, Bern University Hospital (Inselspital) and University Bern, Switzerland

ELENA WENZ, MD
Department of Neurology, Bern University Hospital (Inselspital) and University Bern, Switzerland

PAULA G. WILLIAMS, PhD
Department of Psychology, University of Utah, Salt Lake City, Utah, USA

HOLGER WOEHRLE, MD
Lungenzentrum Ulm, Germany

MARIE-ANGELA WULF, MD, PhD
Department of Neurology, Bern University Hospital (Inselspital) and University Bern, Switzerland

Contents

aim of this review is to offer an overview of how different tests have been used in the field, mapping each test onto a corresponding cognitive domain and propose how to move forward with a suggested cognitive battery of tests covering all major cognitive domains.

Several questionnaires aka patient-reported outcome measures (PROMs) have been developed for specific use in sleep medicine. Some PROMS are "disease-specific," that is, related to a specific sleep disorder, whereas others are generic. These PROMS constitute a valuable add-on to the conventional history taking. They can be used in the areas of research, clinical practice, and quality of health care appraisal. Still, these instruments have inherent limitations, requiring proficient application in the various areas of interest. Disease-specificity includes a risk for nosologic bias that may confound diagnostic and therapeutic results. Future research should provide solutions for shortcomings of presently available questionnaires.

Wearable technology has a history in sleep research dating back to the 1970s. Because modern wearable technology is relatively cheap and widely used by the general population, this represents an opportunity to leverage wearable devices to advance sleep medicine and research. However, there is a lack of published validation studies designed to quantify device performance against accepted gold standards, especially across different populations. Recommendations for conducting performance assessments and using wearable devices are now published with the goal of standardizing wearable device implementation and advancing the field.

Sleep health and tracking sleep with contemporary wearables have become more popular. Sleep disorders, in particular, sleep-disordered breathing, have a higher prevalence than estimated previously. Many patients with apnea and hypopnea events suffer whereas others do not report complaints or show cardiovascular consequences. Assessment with wearables may support efforts to distinguish which type of apnea is related to aging and which to cardiovascular comorbidities. Innovative methods offer smart solutions for problems that are insufficiently addressed. Telemedical concepts help bring patients to sleep medicine expertise at an early stage. To use these methods clinically, they must be certified as medical devices.

Sleep in women and men have been studied in several studies with higher prevalence of sleep complaints in women compared with men. Several factors can affect sleep and could be argued to contribute to sex and gender differences in general sleep. There are no differences in guidelines when measuring sleep in women but several sleep assessment tools have been validated or compared between sexes. Because there is still a lack of knowledge on sleep measurements in women, the present review aimed to produce an overview of the current knowledge of objective and subjective sleep measurements in women.

Sleep Measurement in Children—Are We on the Right Track? 649

Barbara Gnidovec Stražišar

Sleep plays a critical role in the development of healthy children. Detecting sleep and sleep disorders and the effectiveness of interventions for improving sleep in children require valid sleep measures. Assessment of sleep in children, in particular infants and young children, can be a quite challenging task. Many subjective and objective methods are available to evaluate various aspects of sleep in childhood, each with their strengths and limitations. None can, however, replace the importance of thorough clinical interview with detailed history and clinical examination by a sleep specialist.

Measuring Sleep, Wakefulness, and Circadian Functions in Neurologic Disorders 661

Markus H. Schmidt, Martijn P.J. Dekkers, Sébastien Baillieul, Jasmine Jendoubi, Marie-Angela Wulf, Elena Wenz, Livia Fregolente, Albrecht Vorster, Oriella Gnarra, and Claudio L.A. Bassetti

Neurologic disorders impact the ability of the brain to regulate sleep, wake, and circadian functions, including state generation, components of state (such as rapid eye movement sleep muscle atonia, state transitions) and electroencephalographic microarchitecture. At its most extreme, extensive brain damage may even prevent differentiation of sleep stages from wakefulness (eg, status dissociatus). Given that comorbid sleep-wake-circadian disorders are common and can adversely impact the occurrence, evolution, and management of underlying neurologic conditions, new technologies for long-term monitoring of neurologic patients may potentially usher in new diagnostic strategies and optimization of clinical management.

Preface
Improving Sleep Measurements for the Future

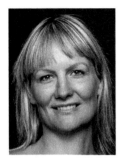

Erna Sif Arnardottir, PhD
Editor

The field of sleep is at a crossroads. Experts in sleep medicine and sleep research are calling out for new methods for both the diagnosis and treatment of different sleep disorders. We are realizing that the current state-of-the-art sleep measurement is not sufficient. We need to raise the bar and employ emerging technology to the fullest for the benefit of the numerous patients with sleep problems. This challenge is highlighted in the 10 excellent reviews in this issue on different aspects of sleep measurements. Importantly, both objective and subjective ways to measure sleep are discussed, as the role of the subjective sleep measurement is equally important as the objective one.

The need for sleep studies has increased exponentially in recent years as awareness for the importance of a good night's sleep has exploded among the general population and health care staff. Therefore, the current gold standard of in-laboratory polysomnography must be challenged and, in many cases, be moved to self-applied home sleep recordings to decrease the long waiting lists, workload, and costs of each sleep study. The heavy manual labor of scoring each sleep study also must be shortened for the same reasons. Finally, new parameters informing us better about the treatment need of individual patients than the current parameters are desperately needed. The role of interdisciplinary work, that is, working with experts in machine learning to move beyond the current state-of-the-art, is paramount to achieve these needed changes and to get more from sleep recordings than we currently do.

The role of daytime functioning, including objective cognitive performance and subjective measurements or patient-reported outcomes, is also of great importance. This field of sleep measurements needs substantial improvement to further understand how people are affected by sleep issues and to enhance patient care as reviewed in this issue. The role of wearable and digital health technology for our patient populations is another hot topic. The potential of this technology to complement traditional health care and research methods is huge. Sleep experts as a whole need to take advantage of this to the best of their abilities and perform the relevant research studies to validate their role. Finally, three different subgroups of patients are studied in more detail: women, children, and patients with neurologic disorders, to emphasize the need for different measurement tools and validations of such tools for different patient groups.

One size does indeed not fit all. Personalized sleep medicine, different treatment options as well as predictive, preventive, and participatory elements are all needed to push the boundaries of the sleep field. It is time for a revolution of sleep measurements!

Erna Sif Arnardottir, PhD
Reykjavik University Sleep Institute
School of Technology
Reykjavik University
Menntavegi 1
102 Reykjavik, Iceland

E-mail address:
ernasifa@ru.is

Sleep Med Clin 16 (2021) xiii
https://doi.org/10.1016/j.jsmc.2021.09.001
1556-407X/21/© 2021 Published by Elsevier Inc.

Self-Applied Home Sleep Recordings
The Future of Sleep Medicine

Henri Korkalainen, PhD[a,b,*,1], Sami Nikkonen, PhD[a,b,1],
Samu Kainulainen, PhD[a,b], Amit Krishna Dwivedi, PhD[a,b],
Sami Myllymaa, PhD[a,b], Timo Leppänen, PhD[a,b,c], Juha Töyräs, PhD[a,c,d]

KEYWORDS

- Sleep disorders • Home sleep recordings • Machine learning • Deep learning
- Electroencephalography • Photoplethysmography • Wearables • Medical devices

KEY POINTS

- Polysomnography is expensive, requires substantial labor, and has limited availability; thus, there is an increasing need for simple home-based recordings.
- Advancements in machine learning and artificial intelligence allow automatic analysis of sleep recordings; these approaches are already reaching accuracy on par with manual scoring by clinical experts.
- There is immense potential in using wearable sensing solutions for screening and long-term monitoring of sleep disorders. Combining simple screening devices with automatic analysis would enable cost-efficient monitoring over multiple nights.
- The pulse oximeter is one of the most potential devices to act as an efficient and accurate standalone screening device. Automatic analysis approaches could be easily adapted to all home-based sleep recordings.
- In some complex cases, simplified recording setups with a reduced electroencephalography montage, pulse oximetry, leg electromyography, and respiratory measurements at home could be used.

INTRODUCTION

Sleep disorders and inadequate sleep are quickly becoming a substantial global health problem. Poor sleep induces a major economical and social burden owing to direct health care costs, loss of productivity, and increased risk of accidents and traffic crashes.[1] Meanwhile, sleep disorders have an increasingly high prevalence. Obstructive sleep apnea (OSA) alone is estimated to affect hundreds of millions of individuals,[2] whereas insomnia symptoms are prevalent in up to one-half of the adult population, with 10% to 15% of the population also suffering from daytime impairment.[3] It is evident that efficient diagnostic practices for sleep medicine are crucial. Owing to the heavy patient inflow and the limited capacity of sleep laboratories, home-based recordings will most likely have an increasing role in the future.

The current gold standard in diagnosing sleep disorders and studying sleep is the type I polysomnography (PSG) conducted at a specialized sleep laboratory. PSG records the electrical activity of the brain (electroencephalography [EEG]), eye

[a] Department of Applied Physics, University of Eastern Finland, PO Box 1627, Kuopio 70211, Finland;
[b] Diagnostic Imaging Center, Kuopio University Hospital, Kuopio, Finland; [c] School of Information Technology and Electrical Engineering, The University of Queensland, Brisbane, Australia; [d] Science Service Center, Kuopio University Hospital, Kuopio, Finland
[1] Co-first authors.
* Corresponding author. Department of Applied Physics, University of Eastern Finland, PO Box 1627, Kuopio 70211, Finland.
E-mail address: henri.korkalainen@uef.fi

Sleep Med Clin 16 (2021) 545–556
https://doi.org/10.1016/j.jsmc.2021.07.003
1556-407X/21/© 2021 Elsevier Inc. All rights reserved.

movements (electro-oculography [EOG]), chin and leg muscle tone (electromyography [EMG]), and cardiac function (electrocardiography [ECG]). In addition, respiratory effort, airflow, blood oxygen saturation, and sleeping position are recorded alongside additional video and audio recordings.[4,5] The signals commonly recorded in modern PSG, the sensors used to record these signals, and the rationale behind the signal inclusion are presented in **Table 1**.

Although type I PSG is the most comprehensive diagnostic method and can be especially useful in the differential diagnosis when multiple sleep disorders are suspected, it has several major limitations and shortcomings. One of the primary drawbacks is high cost. A sleep laboratory staffed with professional sleep technologists is required to conduct the PSG, further increasing complexity and cost.[9] PSG also requires substantial labor from professional sleep technologists because the electrodes and measurement devices must be placed meticulously, the participant must be supervised during the night, and the manual scoring of the recordings is a highly time-consuming process.[10]

Moreover, PSG may not always be fully representative of normal sleep and can suffer from a considerable first night effect, where the unfamiliar environment and complex PSG equipment causes discomfort and stress, disturbing normal sleep.[11,12] The first night effect is very difficult to eliminate completely, even if the sleep laboratory is set up in a more comfortable and less clinical environment, such as in a hotel.[12] Possibly the most effective solution for decreasing or even eliminating the first-night effect is to record sleep for multiple consecutive nights. The benefits of recording sleep over multiple nights are also supported by the fact that there exists significant night-to-night variation in sleep and the severity of some common sleep disorders.[11,13,14] Therefore, it is clear that a single PSG recording may not sufficiently identify all sleep disorders or provide a good representation of a typical night. Nevertheless, owing to the practical constraints discussed elsewhere in this article, only a single monitoring night is almost exclusively used in clinical sleep medicine.[12]

Compared with the full in-laboratory PSG, simpler ambulatory devices are also available for use in sleep diagnostics.[6] The Task Force of the Standards of Practice Committee of the American Sleep Disorder Association has defined 4 monitor types for sleep recording.[5] The requirements for each category are presented in **Table 2**. Type I recording is a standard attended in-laboratory PSG that is recommended for most sleep studies and often required to diagnose complex sleep disorders.[5,15] Type II recording refers to a full PSG setup conducted unattended in a home environment, often without the video and audio recordings. A type III device is an unattended polygraphy device used to diagnose some sleep disorders, for example, OSA. However, it cannot

---

Table 1
The signals included in modern polysomnography (PSG), the commonly used sensor types, and the main diagnostic use of the recorded signals[4–8]

Recording	Sensor Types	Main Diagnostic Use
Airflow	Thermistor, nasal pressure sensor	Respiratory event scoring
Audio	Microphone, piezoelectric sensor	Breathing and snoring sounds
Blood oxygen saturation	Pulse oximeter	Desaturation event scoring
Body position	Accelerometer	Identify positional sleep apnea
Electrical activity of the brain	Cup electrodes	Sleep stage and arousal scoring
Eye movements	Adhesive electrodes, cup electrodes	Sleep staging
Cardiac function	Adhesive electrodes	Heart rate
Muscle tone and leg movements	Adhesive electrodes	Sleep staging and periodic limb movements
Respiratory effort	RIP belts, piezoelectric sensor	Differentiating central, mixed, and obstructive apneas
Video	Video camera	Investigating behavioral patterns and identifying issues in recording

Abbreviation: RIP, respiratory inductance plethysmography.

Table 2
The different sleep monitor types as defined by the Task Force of the Standards of Practice Committee of the American Sleep Disorder Association[5,8,18]

Sleep Study Type	Diagnostic Purpose	Minimum Number of Signals	Required Signals
Type I in-laboratory PSG	Various sleep disorders	8	EEG, EOG, chin EMG, ECG, airflow, respiratory effort, body position, oxygen saturation
Type II unattended PSG	Various sleep disorders	7	EEG, EOG, chin EMG, heart rate, airflow, respiratory effort, oxygen saturation
Type III unattended polygraphy	Mainly sleep apnea	4	Respiratory effort, airflow, heart rate, oxygen saturation
Type IV unattended recording	Mainly monitoring	1	Respiratory effort or airflow or oxygen saturation

This table presents the minimum requirements; however, many modern sleep monitors record more signals.

Abbreviations: ECG, electrocardiography; EEG, electroencephalography; EMG, electromyography; EOG, electrooculography; PSG, polysomnography.

be used to fully replace PSG owing to the lack of EEG, preventing accurate sleep staging and detecting arousals from sleep.[10] Most recording devices that are accepted to be used for sleep disorder diagnosis are of types I through III. Only a few type IV devices, required to record a single channel, are in diagnostic use.

The main advantage of home-based measurements is the capability of the studied individual to sleep in a familiar environment. Moreover, home recordings do not require health care practitioners for active monitoring, thus providing a more cost-efficient option over an in-laboratory PSG.[15] However, ambulatory devices have their limitations, because they generally cannot be used fully independently and thus still require at least some training and set up by a professional. For example, a type II PSG usually requires a sleep technologist to place at least the EEG electrodes and set up the device, which takes approximately an hour of time.[10] Type III devices may be equipped by the studied individual and only guidance is required from health care professionals. However, mistakes made by patients and incorrect use of the devices in unattended conditions lead to greater failure rates and poorer signal quality compared with full in-laboratory PSG.[15,16] This factor, in turn, facilitates an increased need for retesting, therefore mitigating some of the cost benefits of the ambulatory devices over type I PSG.[15,16] Ambulatory devices also suffer from a higher rate of data loss, which can lead to inconclusive results and further necessitate retesting.[17]

The classification of sleep monitoring devices was done more than 2 decades ago and it remains the current official specification.[5] However, there have been massive advancements in sensor, signal analysis, and recording technology after this specification. Therefore, there can be a wide range in capability between devices of the same type. It should also be noted that the American Academy of Sleep Medicine (AASM) has not included this sleep monitor type classification in their scoring manual and only separates between in-laboratory PSG (type I) and home sleep apnea test devices (types II–IV).

It is clear that simpler, more affordable, and fully automatic devices, diagnostic methods, and analytic tools are needed in sleep diagnostics. These new approaches could simultaneously mitigate some of the shortcomings of current diagnostic methods while allowing more widespread screening and diagnosis. This process would in turn enable treatment and its follow-up monitoring for many who are currently suffering from a sleep disorder but are not diagnosed owing to waiting times or limited diagnostic resources. Overall, current technical innovations could be exploited to streamline the diagnostic process and move toward the next-generation self-applied home sleep recordings. Mainly, the advancements in easy-to-use wearable sensors and automated analyses based on artificial intelligence (AI), or more precisely machine learning and deep learning, could allow simpler and more affordable sleep recordings in the future. Elsewhere in this article, we present our views on the future of sleep recordings based on the most recent advancements in sensing technology and AI-based analysis methods.

RECORDING AND SCORING OF SLEEP STAGES

Sleep staging is traditionally performed by manually reviewing the PSG recordings in 30-second segments, called epochs. Each epoch of sleep is scored to 1 of 5 stages: stage W (wakefulness), stage R (REM sleep), and 3 non-REM (NREM) stages (N1, N2, and N3). The most common characteristics of each sleep stage are presented in **Table 3**. Identifying sleep stages is mainly based on EEG, EOG, and chin EMG signal features, patterns, and waveforms. The gold standard of identifying sleep stages requires recordings of 3 EEG channels (F4–M1, C4–M1, and O2–M1,) with 3 additional backup channels (F3–M2, C3–M2, and O1–M2), 2 EOG channels, and a chin-EMG channel.[4] However, it has been reported that using all these recommended channels might not be necessary for accurate sleep staging because other derivations will only lead to slightly different results in sleep stage scoring.[19,20]

Sleep staging is currently only possible from type I and type II PSGs and the sleep architecture remains unknown with other types of sleep recordings. This factor inhibits using types III and IV recording devices when diagnosing most sleep disorders, especially in complex situations with several comorbid sleep disorders. The self-applied type III recordings are most often used in diagnosing OSA because the respiratory events during the night can mostly be identified without the sleep staging. Type III devices are even the preferred diagnostic method for OSA in some health care systems because they are simpler and allow the patient to sleep at home, thus decreasing costs and increasing patient comfort.[21,22] However, the lack of sleep staging and EEG recording leads to an unreliable estimation of OSA severity because some respiratory events require EEG-based arousal detection to be detected accurately.[23] In addition, the total sleep time is important for accurate estimation of OSA severity and if the total recording time is used instead of the total sleep time, OSA severity can be significantly underestimated.[23] Still, the same thresholds are used for defining the OSA severity and choosing the patients for receiving health insurance- or government-subsidized treatment regardless of the diagnostic device type.[24,25] In

Table 3
The common characteristics of sleep stages.[4,8]

Sleep Stage	Characterized by	Clarification
Stage W	Alpha rhythm	Sinusoidal 8–13 Hz activity in EEG
	Eye blinking	Vertical eye movements at a frequency range of 0.5–2 Hz
	High muscle tone	High chin EMG activity
Stage N1	LAMF activity	LAMF EEG activity mostly at 4–7 Hz
	Slow eye movements	Regular, sinusoidal eye movements with a deflection duration of >0.5 s
	Varying muscle tone	Chin EMG activity varies but is generally lower than during wake
Stage N2	K complexes	A sharp wave with both negative and positive components
	Sleep spindles	A train of sinusoidal waves (11–16 Hz) with a duration >0.5 s
	Low EOG, varying EMG	Usually minimal eye movements
		Chin EMG activity varies but is usually lower than during wake
Stage N3	Slow-wave activity	Slow waves (0.5–2 Hz) with an amplitude of >75 µV
	No eye movements	Usually, no visible eye movements and the EOG only displays the same frequencies as the EEG
	Low EMG	Chin EMG activity is usually the lowest of all NREM stages
Stage R	Rapid eye movements	Irregular, sharp eye movements with a deflection duration of <0.5 s
	Low chin muscle tone	EMG activity at the lowest level of all sleep stages
	Transient muscle activity	Short irregular bursts of EMG activity usually with duration of <0.25 s
	Sawtooth waves	Trains of triangular, serrated, 2–6 Hz waves

Abbreviations: ECG, electrocardiography; EEG, electroencephalography; EMG, electromyography; EOG, electrooculography; LAMF, Low-amplitude mixed-frequency; NREM, non-rapid eye movement; PSG, polysomnography; REM, rapid eye movement.

addition, the identification of more specific conditions, such as REM-related OSA, cannot be done without sleep staging. Finally, the differential diagnosis when multiple sleep disorders are suspected is impossible without sleep staging. Therefore, even a simple assessment of sleep architecture would be highly beneficial in home-based measurements.

Self-applicable electrode sets and wearable EEG devices already exist for measuring EEG at home.[20,26–30] These devices do not require any input from a sleep technologist to set up, aside from possibly providing instructions. They usually measure the EEG from the forehead area instead of the crown typically done in 10 to 20 derived systems (**Fig. 1**). For example, a screen-printed self-applicable electrode set has been successfully used in identifying sleep stages with a low failure rate and high correspondence to type I PSG.[20,29] Because the electrode set enables good quality measurements without the need for any skin preparation, it would be well-suited for self-applied home measurements.[31] However, these devices still require manual sleep stage scoring. In addition, because these devices use nonstandard electrode placements, they require rigorous validation before they can be adopted for clinical use. This is because the forehead EEG signals collected from nonstandard locations may not contain exactly the same information as signals from the 10 to 20 system; thus the standard scoring rules may not be applicable as such without adjustments.

The AASM also considers peripheral arterial tonometry (PAT) devices acceptable for estimating sleep time and for the identification of respiratory events.[4] At least one such device, the Watch PAT, is on the market, although the accuracy of the device is not on par with standard home sleep apnea test methods.[32–35]

Recently, there has been an increasing number of consumer-grade wearable devices for assessing sleep quality. These products include devices such as wristbands, smartwatches, and rings for sleep tracking. Despite having suffered from low reliability compared with type I PSG during disordered sleep,[36] there may be the potential to enable the simple and comfortable long-term assessment of sleep architecture in the future. However, rigorous clinical validation and appropriate medical approval processes are certainly needed before any of these can be adapted to diagnostic practices.

With the advancement of machine learning methodology, different solutions capable of identifying sleep stages from simple measurements have been introduced. Machine learning methods have enabled highly accurate sleep staging even based on a single frontal EEG channel, with epoch-by-epoch accuracies as high as 83%.[37–40] In comparison, the interscorer agreement in the AASM interscorer reliability program was reported to be 82.6%.[41] Therefore, these machine learning–based models seem to be already comparable with expert manual scoring. Similar approaches have also been able to provide an estimate of the sleep architecture based on simpler surrogate measurements. For example, ECG measurement has been used successfully in differentiating between sleep and wakefulness.[42–44] Even simpler solutions may be used; for example, a photoplethysmogram (PPG) measured with a pulse oximeter has been shown to be a viable option.[45–48] With deep learning applied to PPG, it has been shown that differentiating between the individual sleep stages is possible with a moderate agreement to manual scoring of PSG (64.1%), and good agreement in differentiating between NREM, REM, and wakefulness (80.1%)[45] (**Fig. 2A**). The PPG-based sleep

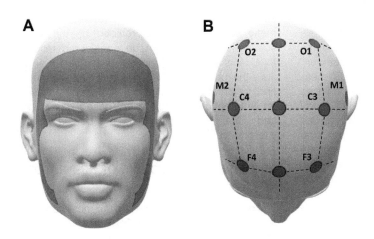

Fig. 1. Forehead/face (*gray*) is a common area to attach self-applicable electrodes used in wearable EEG devices[20,28,30] (*A*). The 10 to 20 system-derived electrode places are used in conventional in-laboratory PSG (*B*).

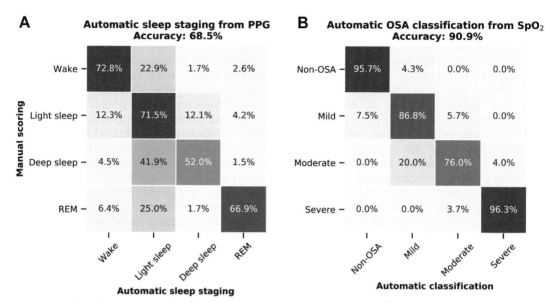

A Automatic sleep staging from PPG
Accuracy: 68.5%

B Automatic OSA classification from SpO$_2$
Accuracy: 90.9%

Fig. 2. Examples of automatic pulse oximetry-based sleep stage classification[45] (*A*) and apnea–hypopnea index (AHI) estimation[53] (*B*) and how they correspond with expert manual scoring. The sleep stages and AHI were automatically determined from the PPG and the blood oxygen saturation (SpO$_2$) signals, respectively. As such, these results highlight what can be already achieved using only a single probe-pulse oximetry measurement instead of the full PSG setup.

staging could be extremely useful, even if not as accurate as EEG-based sleep staging because it only requires a simple pulse oximeter, which is a cheap, easy to use, and reliable sensor that is already integrated into all type I, II, and III recording devices. In addition, it is completely noninvasive and causes minimal disruption to sleep and thus would be highly useful for reduced recording setups such as type III or type IV recordings. Therefore, comparing PPG sleep staging accuracy with the accuracy of full PSG setup may not be always relevant, because it would be only used in situations where EEG recording is not available.

The future of sleep recording at home certainly lies in implementing simple measurement devices capable of identifying sleep stages. Whenever a sensitive and accurate measurement is required, the self-applicable electrode sets would be the most viable option owing to their simple placement and easy comparison with standard EEG measurements. Consumer-grade wearable devices have great potential, but are currently not ready for use in a diagnostic setting before a rigorous clinical validation and medical approval process. Wearable devices would provide an even simpler setup compared with single-use self-applicable electrode sets and would enable convenient over consecutive nights. Although they may be more prone to failed measurements and poor placement, long-term monitoring could make up for these limitations. Finally, whenever the information

on the total sleep time and a rough division to NREM, REM, and wakefulness are sufficient, the surrogate measures to EEG for sleep staging are the most viable option. For example, PPG is already recorded during practically all home-based sleep measurements and would not require any additional sensors to enable differentiation of sleep stages.

Most sleep analysis software, such as Noxturnal (Nox system, Nox Medical, Reykjavik, Iceland), RemLogic (Embla/Embletta systems, Natus, Broomfiled, CO), and Sleepware 3G (Philips Alice system, Philips, Amsterdam, the Netherlands), also allows automatic sleep staging and respiratory event scoring. However, the accuracy of these methods varies and, in most cases, is not thoroughly tested or reported. Therefore, the automatic scoring methods provided by the sleep scoring software cannot be considered reliable for clinical use without manual correction. In addition, the position of AASM is still that diagnosis and treatment decisions cannot be only based on automatic methods or AI-based algorithms and the raw data must be manually interpreted.[49,50]

RECORDING AND SCORING OF RESPIRATORY EVENTS

The diagnosis of OSA is among the most common reasons for conducting a PSG because it has been estimated that as much as one-half of the adult population is afflicted by OSA according to current clinical standards.[2] OSA is a nocturnal breathing disorder characterized by frequent obstructions in the upper airways during sleep. These obstructions lead to either complete (apnea) or partial (hypopnea) cessations in breathing, called respiratory events.[4] The diagnosis of OSA is primarily based on the number of apnea and hypopnea events per hour of sleep, called the apnea–hypopnea index (AHI), which determines the severity of OSA.[4] More precisely, OSA is diagnosed if the AHI is 5 or more with associated signs or symptoms of sleepiness or if the AHI is 15 or more, even without any symptoms.[4,51] Therefore, the diagnosis of OSA requires the detection of respiratory events from PSG signals. This process is currently done manually by annotating the signals using visual scoring rules, which is very time consuming. Although most recording software provides initial built-in automated scoring, it is not meant for final diagnosis and still needs to be corrected manually and evaluated. These factors make respiratory event scoring currently very laborious and therefore also expensive.[10]

A wide variety of automatic classification methods for the detection of OSA exist.[52] Most of these methods are not capable of scoring individual events or even estimating the AHI, making them unable to accurately evaluate the OSA severity.[52] However, recent studies have shown that, by using machine learning methods, an extremely accurate and fully automatic estimation of the AHI is possible based solely on the oxygen saturation signal.[53] For example, greater than 90% accuracy in OSA severity estimation with a median AHI error of less than 1 has been reported in an home sleep apnea test dataset using the 4% desaturation criteria for hypopnea scoring[53] (**Fig. 2**B). Similar results have also been shown in patients with cerebrovascular disease and in large external test populations indicating good generalizability and robustness of these methods.[53,54] A further advantage of these methods is that they only require the blood oxygen saturation recording during the night; thus, they can be applied easily to all types of PSG or home sleep monitoring devices, because the oxygen saturation is acquired with a pulse oximeter, which is already included in all type I, II, and III devices. As mentioned elsewhere in this article, the pulse oximeter is a simple and easy-to-use sensor to that requires no end-user calibration or complex set up. Therefore, the pulse oximetry–based OSA severity estimation could be especially suitable for large-scale screening of OSA and in various settings of scientific research.

Although the pulse oximetry–based methods are well-suited for tasks such as large-scale screening for OSA, they are so far only able to provide estimates of the AHI and OSA severity and cannot be used to diagnose more specific variants of sleep apnea, for example, central sleep apnea, supine dominant or isolated OSA, or REM-related OSA. Therefore, these automatic methods cannot be compared directly with standard manual respiratory event scoring or used for detailed respiratory event analysis. However, this kind of fully automatic respiratory event scoring based on machine learning methods has also been recently shown possible.[8] The automatic respiratory event scoring has been reported with an agreement of 88.9% ($\kappa = 0.728$) with manual scoring, which is very close to the interscorer agreement reported by the AASM interscorer reliability program (93.9%; $\kappa = 0.92$).[8,41] Therefore, automatic machine learning–based scoring could also be applied for comprehensive respiratory event scoring when it is required, with an accuracy that is near human expert scoring. One disadvantage of this method is that the machine learning model also requires respiratory effort and airflow signals in addition to the blood oxygen saturation, and therefore requires a more complex recording setup.[8] However, all of these signals are relatively easy to record and are present in all type I, II, and III sleep monitors. Therefore, this method could be best suited for decreasing the manual scoring workload for recording setups where more information on the respiratory events, other than their frequency, is needed.

As with sleep staging and other sleep disorders, there is also considerable night-to-night variation in OSA severity.[11,13] Thus, multiple night studies could greatly increase the accuracy of the OSA severity evaluation as easy-to-record signals with accompanying automatic analysis could be simply conducted for multiple consecutive nights with minimal additional cost or resources. This process would simultaneously eliminate the first night effect of sleeping with an unfamiliar and uncomfortable recording setup and the random night-to-night variation in sleep patterns that is always present.

IDENTIFYING AROUSALS FROM SLEEP

Arousals from sleep are defined as an abrupt shift in EEG frequencies lasting for more than 3 seconds.[4] Therefore, identifying these requires an EEG recording. Moreover, because the arousals are further differentiated to spontaneous arousals, respiratory arousals, respiratory effort-related arousals, and periodic limb movement arousals, these events require additional measurements, that is, breathing signals and leg EMG signals. Currently, these all are only included in type I and type II recordings.

Similar to sleep staging, the automatic identification of arousals has been conducted based on PSG recordings.[55–57] In 2018, there was a Physio-Net/Computing in Cardiology Challenge to develop an automatic arousal detection software.[55] The winning approach relied on deep learning using EEGs, EOGs, chin EMGs, a respiratory inductance plethysmography belt, oxygen saturation, and airflow signals and achieved reasonable accuracy.[56] Besides requiring a comprehensive measurement setup from a full PSG, the arousal identification only relied on classifying 10-second epochs into arousal or not arousal instead of accurately identifying the actual starting and ending times of the arousals. Aside from these methods, arousal identification has been conducted from ECG recording with promising results.[57] Therefore, there is the potential to conduct automatic detection of arousals in a clinical setting, both from signals recorded during a PSG and from simpler measurements such as PPG. Arousal identification would be crucial to assess sleep fragmentation and in the diagnosis of OSA, because this process would allow for the identification of hypopneas related to arousals. However, more research is warranted before the simpler approaches can be applied in routine clinical practice as scoring of arousals suffers from a relatively low agreement, even between manual scorers evidenced by reported arousal index intraclass correlation of as low as 0.54.[58,59]

IDENTIFYING MOVEMENTS, SNORING, AND CARDIAC EVENTS

Detecting limb movement events is essential for assessing the presence of periodic limb movements and differentiating between different arousals types. The automatic detection of limb movements has also been successfully conducted from leg EMGs relying on deep learning.[60] However, leg EMG recordings are not consistently included in home-based measurements. Thus, AI-based algorithms could be the solution for identifying limb movements from surrogate measures. Potential alternatives include activity-based measurements and position sensors.

Identifying snoring is mostly done based on audio recordings, which can also be conducted automatically.[61,62] Implementing a simple recording of audio to home sleep recordings is straigthforward and can be done, for example, with an ambient microphone or a microphone placed over the trachea. These devices could be accompanied by automatic analyses to easily assess the snoring tendency, which is often also related to OSA. However, in microphone-based snoring detection, it can sometimes be difficult to isolate background noise or bed partner's snoring from the recording, which complicates accurate snoring detection.

The detection of cardiac events conventionally relies on the ECG signal. However, the PPG has immense potential to function as a surrogate for ECG.[63–66] Even though PPG is not a direct measure of the electrical functioning of the heart, the pulse rate and pulse rate variability metrics correlate well with those derived from ECG.[64] Furthermore, computational solutions for PPG-based atrial fibrillation, ectopic complexes, and extrasystole detection exist.[63,65,66] However, these methods warrant further studies on their usability as a part of routine sleep recordings.

THE LIMITATIONS OF HOME RECORDINGS

Home sleep recordings have certain limitations that may be difficult to overcome completely and therefore likely cannot fully replace in-laboratory PSG. For example, in-laboratory PSG often incorporates a video recording of the night. This information is especially crucial when diagnosing disorders such as parasomnias, behavioral nighttime disorders, or nocturnal epilepsy. Diagnosing these entities in a home environment would either require a portable night-vision video recording device with sufficient quality or other surrogate measurements capable of reliably assessing nighttime behaviors. These devices could potentially include sonar-based solutions or accelerometers directly measuring the activity or movement of the individual, with accompanying algorithms for automatic analysis. Moreover, some sleep studies, such as multiple sleep latency testing or the maintenance of wakefulness test, cannot be conducted at home in their current form. Therefore, an accurate objective assessment of daytime sleepiness still requires an in-laboratory recording. Finally, many devices are still relatively difficult to use. Thus, more development work needs to be conducted to improve their usability and make them suitable for all individuals, regardless of factors such as mental status or age.

SUMMARY

Sleep disorders are a global health burden and more efficient diagnostic practices are sorely needed. Home sleep recordings with accompanying AI-based automatic analysis approaches have immense potential to resolve the increasing patient inflows. The specific conclusions related to the future of home sleep recordings are as follows:

1. AI-based sleep staging and OSA severity estimation are already highly accurate and nearly on par with manual scoring. Thus, night-to-night variation, the first night effect, and incorrect use of devices already cause greater uncertainty in the diagnosis than the current automatic analysis methods. As such, the accuracy of these methods is no longer the limiting issue for their adoption and a lack of understanding and trust likely play a much greater role. However, these trust concerns are not entirely unfounded; there is a clear lack of large-scale multicenter validation studies, which are certainly needed before adopting any automatic method for general clinical use.

2. Once validated, the automatic analysis methods could considerably improve the diagnostics of sleep disorders because the automatic methods would not only decrease the workload related to manual scoring, but also make the analysis more consistent and improve the overall accuracy and ease of comparison.

3. Simpler recording setups would be highly useful for screening and assisting in the diagnosis of many sleep disorders. Cheap and easy-to-use recording devices could increase the availability of recordings and enable diagnosis and follow-up of treatment for more individuals. Simpler measurement setups would simultaneously be more comfortable and impose a lesser disruption to sleep. Thus, they could allow obtaining a more reliable representation of natural sleep.

4. Combining automatic AI-based analysis and simple screening devices would enable simple and cost-efficient monitoring over multiple consecutive nights. This practice would minimize the first night effect and the effect of night-to-night variability and release the limited resources of sleep specialists from manual scoring to other tasks.

5. Based on the current research, we consider that pulse oximeter recording, including the PPG and blood oxygen saturation, has the most potential for simple and cost-efficient yet accurate screening of sleep disorders. A pulse oximeter is cheap and easy to use, requires no calibration or difficult setup, and can be used multiple times with no preparation or a need to replace single-use parts such as electrodes. Furthermore, it is fully noninvasive and causes minimal disruption to sleep. These factors make it an ideal sensor for continuous long-term and multi-night recordings. Finally, and most importantly, the measured signals (oxygen saturation and PPG) are extremely information rich and can be alone used to automatically evaluate sleep stages and the severity of OSA with high accuracy (see **Fig. 1**).[45,53]

6. For more complex sleep disorders and specialized analysis, simplified self-applied recording setups with reduced EEG, pulse oximetry, leg EMG, and respiratory measurements could be used. The signals recorded by the simplified devices could still be scored using automatic machine learning-based methods. Traditional type I PSG could be reserved for only those cases that cannot be reliably studied and diagnosed otherwise.

CLINICS CARE POINTS

- In-laboratory PSG is the gold standard method but suffers from high costs, limited availability, and laborsome manual analysis.
- Home recordings are well-suited especially for screening purposes and follow-up monitoring.
- In the future, simpler home recording devices alongside fully automatic analysis have massive potential for sleep disorder diagnostics.
- Current machine learning–based automatic scoring methods can already be considered as accurate as manual scoring; however, more comprehensive validation in heterogeneous populations is needed before widespread clinical adoption.
- Home recordings cannot fully replace the in-laboratory PSG in complex situations or when multiple sleep disorders are suspected.

ACKNOWLEDGMENTS

The authors thank Matias Rusanen for his invaluable assistance in preparing the figures.

DISCLOSURE

This study was financially supported by the European Union's Horizon 2020 research and innovation program under grant agreement no. 965417, NordForsk (NordSleep project 90,458-06111) via Business Finland (5133/31/2018), the Research Committee of the Kuopio University Hospital Catchment Area for the State Research Funding (5041767, 5041768, 5041794, 5041797, 5041798, and 5041803), the Academy of Finland (323536), Tampere Tuberculosis Foundation, Päivikki and Sakari Sohlberg Foundation, Finnish Cultural Foundation – North Savo Regional Fund, and The

Research Foundation of the Pulmonary Diseases. The authors declare no conflicts of interest.

REFERENCES

1. Hillman D, Mitchell S, Streatfeild J, et al. The economic cost of inadequate sleep. Sleep 2018;41(8): zsy083.

2. Benjafield A, Ayas NT, Eastwood PR, et al. Estimation of the global prevalence and burden of obstructive sleep apnoea: a literature-based analysis. Lancet Respir Med 2019;7(8):687–98.

3. Schutte-Rodin S, Broch L, Buysse D, et al. Clinical Guideline for the evaluation and Management of chronic insomnia in adults. J Clin Sleep Med 2008; 4(5):487–504.

4. Berry RB, Albertario CL, Harding SM, et al. The AASM manual for the scoring of sleep and associated events: rules, terminology and technical specifications. Version 2.5. Darien (IL): American Academy of Sleep Medicine; 2018.

5. Ferber R, Millman R, Coppola M, et al. ASDA standards of practice: portable recording in the assessment of obstructive sleep apnea. Sleep 1994;17(4): 378–92.

6. Collop NA, Anderson WMD, Boehlecke B, et al. Clinical guidelines for the use of unattended portable monitors in the diagnosis of obstructive sleep apnea in adult patients. J Clin Sleep Med 2007;3(7):737–47.

7. Bianchi MT. Sleep devices: wearables and nearables, informational and interventional, consumer and clinical. Metabolism 2018;84:99–108.

8. Nikkonen S, Korkalainen H, Leino A, et al. Automatic respiratory event scoring in obstructive sleep apnea using a long short-term memory neural network. IEEE J Biomed Heal Inform 2021. https://doi.org/10.1109/JBHI.2021.3064694.

9. Punjabi NM. The epidemiology of adult obstructive sleep apnea. Proc Am Thorac Soc 2008;5(2): 136–43.

10. Fischer J, Dogas Z, Bassetti CL, et al. Standard procedures for adults in accredited sleep medicine centres in Europe. J Sleep Res 2012;21(4):357–68.

11. Newell J, Mairesse O, Verbanck P, et al. Is a one-night stay in the lab really enough to conclude? First-night effect and night-to-night variability in polysomnographic recordings among different clinical population samples. Psychiatry Res 2012;200(2–3): 795–801.

12. Hutchison KN, Song Y, Wang L, et al. Analysis of sleep parameters in patients with obstructive sleep apnea studied in a hospital vs. a hotel-based sleep center. J Clin Sleep Med 2008;4(2):119–22.

13. Bittencourt LRA, Suchecki D, Peres C, et al. The variability of the apnoea-hypopnoea index. J Sleep Res 2001;10(3):245–51.

14. Miettinen T, Myllymaa K, Hukkanen T, et al. Home polysomnography reveals a first-night effect in patients with low sleep bruxism activity. J Clin Sleep Med 2018;14(8):1377–86.

15. Golpe R, Jimenéz A, Carpizo R. Home sleep studies in the assessment of sleep apnea/hypopnea syndrome. Chest 2002;122(4):1156–61.

16. Whittle AT, Finch SP, Mortimore IL, et al. Use of home sleep studies for diagnosis of the sleep apnoea/hypopnoea syndrome. Pneumologie 1998;52(8):467.

17. Ahmed M, Patel NP, Rosen I. Portable monitors in the diagnosis of obstructive sleep apnea. Chest 2007;132(5):1672–7.

18. Chesson AL, Berry RB, Pack A. Practice parameters for the use of portable monitoring devices in the investigation of suspected obstructive sleep apnea in adults. Sleep 2003;26(7):907–13.

19. Ruehland WR, O'Donoghue FJ, Pierce RJ, et al. The 2007 AASM recommendations for EEG electrode placement in polysomnography: impact on sleep and cortical arousal scoring. Sleep 2011;34(1):73–81.

20. Myllymaa S, Muraja-Murro A, Westeren-Punnonen S, et al. Assessment of the suitability of using a forehead EEG electrode set and chin EMG electrodes for sleep staging in polysomnography. J Sleep Res 2016;25(6):636–45.

21. Flemons WW, Douglas NJ, Kuna ST, et al. Access to diagnosis and treatment of patients with suspected sleep apnea. Am J Respir Crit Care Med 2004; 169(6):668–72.

22. Arnardottir ES, Verbraecken J, Gonçalves M, et al. Variability in recording and scoring of respiratory events during sleep in Europe: a need for uniform standards. J Sleep Res 2016;25(2):144–57.

23. Bianchi MT, Goparaju B. Potential underestimation of sleep apnea severity by at-home kits: rescoring in-laboratory polysomnography without sleep staging. J Clin Sleep Med 2017;13(4):551–5.

24. American Academy of Sleep Medicine. Sleep-related breathing disorders in adults : recommendations for syndrome definition and measurement techniques in clinical research. Sleep 1999;22(5):662–89.

25. Korkalainen H, Töyräs J, Nikkonen S, et al. Mortality-risk-based apnea–hypopnea index thresholds for diagnostics of obstructive sleep apnea. J Sleep Res 2019;28(6):1–7.

26. Levendowski DJ, Ferini-Strambi L, Gamaldo C, et al. The accuracy, night-To-night variability, and stability of frontopolar sleep electroencephalography biomarkers. J Clin Sleep Med 2017;13(6):791–803.

27. Younes M, Soiferman M, Thompson W, et al. Performance of a new portable wireless sleep monitor. J Clin Sleep Med 2017;13(2):245–58.

28. Arnal PJ, Thorey V, Debellemaniere E, et al. The Dreem Headband compared to polysomnography for electroencephalographic signal acquisition and sleep staging. Sleep 2020;43(11):1–13.

29. Miettinen T, Myllymaa K, Westeren-Punnonen S, et al. Success rate and technical quality of home polysomnography with self-applicable electrode set in Subjects with possible sleep bruxism. IEEE J Biomed Heal Inform 2018;22(4):1124–32.

30. Kainulainen S, Korkalainen H, Sigurðardóttir S, et al. Comparison of EEG Signal Characteristics Between Polysomnography and Self Applied Somnography Setup in a Pediatric Cohort. IEEE Access 2021. vol. 9. p. 110916-110926.

31. Kalevo L, Miettinen T, Leino A, et al. Effect of Sweating on electrode-skin Contact Impedances and Artifacts in EEG recordings with various screen-printed Ag/Agcl electrodes. IEEE Access 2020;8:50934–43.

32. Hedner J, White DP, Malhotra A, et al. Sleep staging based on autonomic signals: a multi-center validation study. J Clin Sleep Med 2011;7(3):301–6.

33. Zou D, Grote L, Peker Y, et al. Validation a portable monitoring device for sleep apnea diagnosis in a population based cohort using synchronized home polysomnography. Sleep 2006;29(3):367–74.

34. Choi JH, Lee B, Lee JY, et al. Validating the Watch-PAT for diagnosing obstructive sleep apnea in adolescents. J Clin Sleep Med 2018;14(10):1741–7.

35. Pang KP, Gourin CG, Terris DJ. A comparison of polysomnography and the WatchPAT in the diagnosis of obstructive sleep apnea. Otolaryngol Head Neck Surg 2007;137(4):665–8.

36. Liang Z, Chapa Martell MA. Validity of consumer activity wristbands and wearable EEG for measuring overall sleep parameters and sleep Structure in Free-Living conditions. J Healthc Inform Res 2018; 2(1–2):152–78.

37. Korkalainen H, Aakko J, Nikkonen S, et al. Accurate deep learning-based sleep staging in a clinical population with suspected obstructive sleep apnea. IEEE J Biomed Heal Inform 2019. https://doi.org/10.1109/JBHI.2019.2951346.

38. Mousavi S, Afghah F, Acharya UR. SleepEEGNet: automated sleep stage scoring with sequence to sequence deep learning approach. PLoS One 2019;14(5):e0216456.

39. Phan H, Andreotti F, Cooray N, et al. Joint classification and Prediction CNN Framework for automatic sleep stage classification. IEEE Trans Biomed Eng 2019;66(5):1285–96.

40. Phan H, Mikkelsen K, Chén OY, et al. Personalized automatic sleep staging with single-night data: a pilot study with kl-divergence regularization. Physiol Meas 2020;41(6):064004.

41. Rosenberg RS, Van Hout S. The American Academy of Sleep Medicine inter-scorer reliability program: respiratory events. J Clin Sleep Med 2014;10(4):447–54.

42. Li Q, Li Q, Liu C, et al. Deep learning in the cross-time frequency domain for sleep staging from a single-lead electrocardiogram. Physiol Meas 2018; 39(12):124005.

43. Fonseca P, Long X, Radha M, et al. Sleep stage classification with ECG and respiratory effort. Physiol Meas 2015;36(10):2027–40.

44. Willemen T, Van Deun D, Verhaert V, et al. An evaluation of cardiorespiratory and movement features with respect to sleep-stage classification. IEEE J Biomed Heal Inform 2014;18(2):661–9.

45. Korkalainen H, Aakko J, Duce B, et al. Deep learning enables sleep staging from photoplethysmogram for patients with suspected sleep apnea. Sleep 2020; 43(11):1–10.

46. Fonseca P, Weysen T, Goelema MS, et al. Validation of photoplethysmography-based sleep staging compared with polysomnography in healthy middle-aged adults. Sleep 2017;40(7). https://doi.org/10.1093/sleep/zsx097.

47. Beattie Z, Oyang Y, Statan A, et al. Estimation of sleep stages in a healthy adult population from optical plethysmography and accelerometer signals. Physiol Meas 2017;38(11):1968–79.

48. Dehkordi P, Garde A, Dumont GA, et al. Sleep/wake classification using cardiorespiratory features extracted from photoplethysmogram. Comput Cardiol (2010) 2016;43:1021–4.

49. Rosen IM, Kirsch DB, Carden KA, et al. Clinical use of a home sleep apnea test: an updated American Academy of Sleep Medicine position statement. J Clin Sleep Med 2018;14(12):2075–7.

50. Goldstein CA, Berry RB, Kent DT, et al. Artificial intelligence in sleep medicine: an American Academy of Sleep Medicine position statement. J Clin Sleep Med 2020;16(4):605–7.

51. American Academy of Sleep Medicine. International classification of sleep disorders. 3rd edition. Darien, IL: American Academy of Sleep Medicine; 2014.

52. Uddin MB, Chow CM, Su SW. Classification methods to detect sleep apnea in adults based on respiratory and oximetry signals: a systematic review. Physiol Meas 2018;39(3). https://doi.org/10.1088/1361-6579/aaafb8.

53. Nikkonen S, Afara IO, Leppänen T, et al. Artificial neural network analysis of the oxygen saturation signal enables accurate diagnostics of sleep apnea. Sci Rep 2019;9:1–9.

54. Leino A, Nikkonen S, Kainulainen S, et al. Neural network analysis of nocturnal SpO2 signal enables easy screening of sleep apnea in patients with acute cerebrovascular disease. Sleep Med 2020. https://doi.org/10.1016/j.sleep.2020.12.032.

55. Ghassemi MM, Moody BE, Lehman LWH, et al. The PhysioNet/Computing in Cardiology Challenge 2018. Comput Cardiol (2010) 2018;2018:20–3.

56. Howe-Patterson M, Pourbabaee B, Benard F. Automated detection of sleep arousals from polysomnography data using a dense convolutional neural network. Comput Cardiol (2010) 2018;2018:1–4. https://doi.org/10.22489/CinC.2018.232.

57. Li A, Chen S, Quan SF, et al. A deep learning-based algorithm for detection of cortical arousal during sleep. Sleep 2020;43(12):1–10.

58. Drinnan MJ, Murray A, Griffiths CJ, et al. Interobserver variability in recognizing arousal in respiratory sleep disorders. Am J Respir Crit Care Med 1998;158(2):358–62.

59. Whitney CW, Gottlieb DJ, Redline S, et al. Reliability of scoring respiratory disturbance indices and sleep staging. Sleep 1998;21(7):749–57.

60. Biswal S, Sun H, Goparaju B, et al. Expert-level sleep scoring with deep neural networks. J Am Med Inform Assoc 2018;25(12):1643–50.

61. Azarbarzin A, Moussavi ZMK. Automatic and unsupervised snore sound extraction from respiratory sound signals. IEEE Trans Biomed Eng 2011;58(5):1156–62.

62. Swarnkar VR, Abeyratne UR, Sharan RV. Automatic picking of snore events from overnight breath sound recordings. Proc Annu Int Conf IEEE Eng Med Biol Soc EMBS 2017;2822–5. https://doi.org/10.1109/EMBC.2017.8037444.

63. Pereira T, Tran N, Gadhoumi K, et al. Photoplethysmography based atrial fibrillation detection: a review. Npj Digit Med 2020;3(1). https://doi.org/10.1038/s41746-019-0207-9.

64. Gil E, Orini M, Bailón R, et al. Photoplethysmography pulse rate variability as a surrogate measurement of heart rate variability during non-stationary conditions. Physiol Meas 2010;31(9):1271–90.

65. Saritas T, Greber R, Venema B, et al. Non-invasive evaluation of coronary heart disease in patients with chronic kidney disease using photoplethysmography. Clin Kidney J 2019;12(4):538–45.

66. Drijkoningen L, Lenaerts F, Van Der Auwera J, et al. Validation of a smartphone based photoplethysmographic beat detection algorithm for normal and ectopic complexes. Comput Cardiol (2010) 2014;41:845–8.

Improving Machine Learning Technology in the Field of Sleep

Jacky Mallett, PhD[a],*, Erna Sif Arnardottir, PhD[b,c,1]

KEYWORDS

- Sleep apnea • Deep learning • Polysomnography • Sleep staging

KEY POINTS

- Apnea-hypopnea index (AHI) scoring, currently used for obstructive sleep apnea diagnosis, may underestimate and overestimate the severity of the disease.
- Machine learning research should avoid merging datasets scored using different versions of the AHI and other sleep event standards and clearly state which standards were used.
- Researchers should examine base assumptions in existing scoring and analysis in light of new technology and much larger dataset availability.

INTRODUCTION

Recent advances in machine learning together with equally dramatic advances in the sensitivity and accuracy of monitoring equipment have been rightly heralded for their potential in improving medical diagnosis. Not only can extremely detailed data be collected from a single patient, but it is now increasingly practical to create datasets containing information from thousands of individuals. Until the recent introduction of home monitoring equipment, sleep data in particular were difficult and expensive to collect in the laboratory, but this is changing. Although these developments offer considerable potential, there are equally significant obstacles, ranging from the simple practical challenges of working with large datasets[a1] to the problem of working with current medical diagnostics that contain a set of subtle traps for medical and machine learning research.

The aim of this article is to examine the challenges presented to automatic analysis for obstructive sleep apnea (OSA) by the existing scoring standards and diagnostic criteria. Known uncertainties circling around the recording and scoring of OSA severity, which the authors summarize later, can interact poorly with modern approaches to machine learning, especially those using black box techniques based on deep learning. The goal of this article is to provide guidance for researchers striving to resolve these issues.

HOW OBSTRUCTIVE SLEEP APNEA IS DIAGNOSED

OSA is characterized by repeated temporary breathing cessations during sleep due to upper airway closure, typically accompanied by intermittent loud snoring. These respiratory events can lower the blood oxygen level repeatedly

Funding: The Icelandic Research Fund (174067-053, 175256-0611) and NordForsk grant no.90458.
[a] Department of Computer Science, Reykjavik University, Menntavegur 1, Reykjavik 102, Iceland; [b] Reykjavik University Sleep Institute, Reykjavik University, Reykjavik, Iceland; [c] Internal Medicine Services, Landspitali–The National University Hospital of Iceland, Reykjavik, Iceland
[1] Present address: Menntavegi 1, 102 Reykjavik, Iceland.
* Corresponding author.
E-mail address: jacky@ru.is

[a]Some are mundane. Internet transfer times vary considerably, and as a rough rule of thumb, 500 GB will take at least 11 hours at 100 Mbps to ~1 hour at 1Gbit/s to transfer, but these times can vary considerably depending on time of day and local Internet provision.

throughout the night, and also cause brief arousals from sleep, interrupting the normal sleep cycle, usually without the awareness of the patient. OSA is considered to be a progressive condition in adults, but it is also found in children, in whom it can present differently.[2] Long-term consequences for the patient are believed to include excessive daytime sleepiness, hypertension, cardiovascular disease, and premature death.[3]

Today, diagnosis of OSA typically involves a sleep study involving all-night monitoring of a range of physiologic signals with a questionnaire on symptoms and comorbidities. The sleep study will typically measure signals such as airflow via nose (and mouth), chest and abdominal movements, blood oxygen level (SpO_2), pulse, position and movements, electrocardiography (ECG), electroencephalography (EEG), electrooculography (EOG), and electromyography of the chin and legs.[4] Sleep studies can be performed in a dedicated sleep laboratory, but increasingly are conducted with portable measurement devices at home, which may then be followed by an in-laboratory sleep laboratory assessment if needed.[5] Home sleep apnea testing (HSAT) is becoming popular worldwide due to its simplicity and low cost, as it allows patients to hook-up the equipment themselves. Currently, most self-applied HSAT performed are without EEG, EOG, and ECG and consequently do not allow detailed sleep assessment, but this is changing.[6] Accompanying HSAT, there has been an explosion in clinical data to be analyzed, as well as a significant increase in the amount of data available for research, creating an urgent need for reliable methods to automatically analyze sleep data.

Reliably and automatically diagnosing sleep data is still a work in progress. Analysis is currently performed manually by sleep scoring professionals with automatic scoring assistance of some signals. It is both labor intensive and highly skilled. Automatic scoring of arousals is poor, so sleep technologists may need to manually count ∼30 to 100 events an hour for severe OSA. The typical workload for scoring a clinical sleep study is about 2 hours,[7] and with the increasing incidence of OSA in the general population this is stressing the availability of the skilled sleep technicians needed to analyse this data.[8]

Many of the existing diagnostic and measurement criteria were first developed in the 1960s, and although they have been updated over time, their base premises have generally not been reexamined against the considerably improved capabilities of twenty-first century devices. The use of a 30-second segment to analyze EEG readings

for example can be traced to the physical size of band printer paper in the 1960s.

Scoring of individual tests is usually performed following guidelines published by the American Academy of Sleep Medicine (AASM), which defines the apnea-hypopnea index (AHI) for assessing the severity of OSA. Originally performed using the Chicago criteria dating from 1999,[9] there is now a detailed scoring manual that has been continuously updated by the AASM since 2007,[4] with both minor and significant changes. The justification for these changes is not always clear. This continuous modification of the standard creates difficulties for both manual and automatic scoring approaches, especially when sleep studies and research that used different versions of the guidelines are compared. An examination across different sleep centers demonstrated that differences between the scoring criteria can have a significant effect on the patient's AHI measurement and whether or not they are offered treatment.[10,11] Use of the AASM is also far from universal. For example, there are significant variations across European sleep centers that not only use different versions of the AASM guidelines but in some cases have developed their own definitions[7]; this also reflects a lack of agreed international standards on scoring, as only the American standards are currently available as a reference.

These uncertainties with scoring, alongside differences in calibration between different physiologic sensors, can interact with modern approaches to machine learning such as those based on deep learning, in unfortunate ways. Superficially the AHI index on which OSA diagnosis is based offers a clear-cut definition for diagnosis, derived from counting the number of breathing cessations (apneas) and periods of reduced airflow (hypopneas) per hour of sleep. However, hypopneas are normally only counted if they are accompanied either by an arousal from sleep or a desaturation of 3% or more, or in some versions 4% or more, desaturation. In the original Chicago criteria, hypopneas could also be counted if a reduction in nasal pressure or flow of greater than 50% occurred without any downstream effects. Superficially these are precise targets that make them ideal for deep learning approaches, which rely on training neural networks against precisely labeled datasets to identify underlying patterns in the data. This, however, rests on the idea that a simplistic absolute score can adequately capture the complex set of physiologic readings required for the diagnosis of sleep disorders, which with OSA in particular is questionable. It also assumes that interscorer reliability is very high, that is, there is little ambiguity in scoring

A **B**

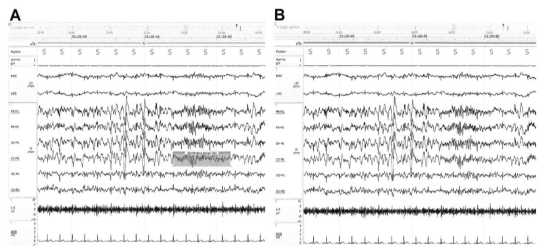

Figure 1. Discrepancies in manual scoring of the same epoch by 2 sleep experts using the same scoring guidelines. (*A*) is scored as sleep stage 1 with an arousal. (*B*) is scored as sleep stage 2 with no arousal.

events, which unfortunately is also not the case (**Fig. 1**).[10]

The AHI itself does not assess duration, depth, or other features of an event in correlation with disease severity, symptoms, or comorbidities. Diagnosis of OSA depends on a simple count of events: mild OSA is defined as 5 to 14.9 events per hour and moderate as 15 to 29.9 and severe OSA as 30 or more respiratory events per hour of sleep independent of their length (**Fig. 2**). The count for severe OSA implies that the patient is having respiratory events at 2-minute frequencies or less. Mathematically this approach seems suspect, because a linear approach is being taken to a nonlinear relationship. Why would 29 events, an event frequency of 2.06 minutes, be considered moderate disease, whereas a 2-minute frequency is classified as severe? At the other extreme with mild OSA, the relatively high error rate with scoring can lead to similarly arbitrary cutoffs, as a relatively small number of events are considered sufficient to diagnose the condition: a minimum 40 events for an 8-hour recording in adults and 8 events in children (AHI $\geq$1 considered mild OSA). Diagnosis of OSA based on the AHI index is not as clear cut as its simple numerical index may make it seem.[12]

THE MECHANISMS OF OBSTRUCTIVE SLEEP APNEA IN A NUTSHELL

The following are believed to be the primary physical mechanisms currently implicated in the long-term impact of OSA on patient health:

(1) OSA's interruption of the normal sleep cycle with repeated arousals and their impact on the patient's autonomous nervous system, increasing sympathetic activity and inflammation, and in particular interfering with deep sleep and rapid eye movement (REM) sleep stages.

(2) The repeated deoxygenation events of the condition causing oxidative stress, sympathetic activity, and inflammation.[3]

The role of other mechanisms such as respiratory effort and snoring are not yet as well understood.[13] When events occur in the sleep cycle may also be important. Some patients experience OSA mainly during the REM sleep stage, or only in the supine position, but because this variation is not included in the diagnostic criteria, their overall AHI is lower than for subjects with events across all sleep stages and positions. For example, studies have shown that OSA events during REM sleep are independently associated with hypertension, increased insulin resistance, and spatial navigational memory impairment, indicating that REM sleep apnea should be investigated further.[14]

Obesity is regarded as one of the strongest risk factors for OSA, and a strong correlation between an increasing AHI and weight gain has been reported over a 5-year period. Although weight gain is a risk factor in the development of OSA, it is also suspected that OSA may lead to increased weight gain, due to the interruption of sleeping patterns, and an associated impact on appetite regulation.[15–17]

Other impacts on health are believed to occur from the physical impact of sustained snoring; this is implicated in the development of carotid atherosclerosis and has been independently

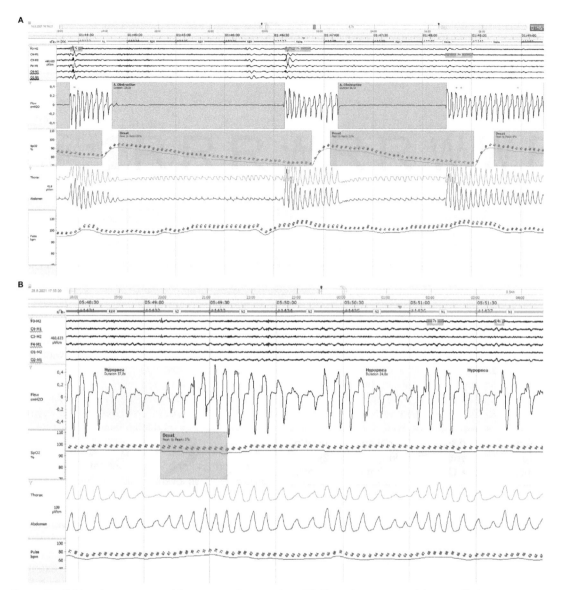

Figure 2. *A*) Very long apneas with a severe desaturation. (*B*) Short hypopneas with a small desaturation or arousals only. All events in panel (*A*) and (*B*) are considered equal in the apnea-hypopnea index and count equally to the severity of the disease in clinical terms.

linked with heavy snoring.[18] A heavy snorer without OSA may therefore experience adverse health effects, but more objective studies are needed, as research to date has been mainly performed with questionnaires.[19]

There is evidence for a potential association between OSA and cancer, particularly in women, with both intermittent hypoxia and sleep fragmentation being suspected as mechanisms. A connection between women with OSA, nocturnal hypoxia, and higher breast cancer rates, but not men, was recently reported.[20] However, the significance level was only $P = .02$ and the actual number of

cancer cases relatively small. With a cutoff for mild AHI of greater than or equal to 5, it is entirely possible that the study itself was affected by the issues described here, as there are significant issues with the categorization of mild AHI due to the proportionally higher impact of errors in sleep scoring for low numbers of events.

Population analysis from large datasets can consequently be challenging to interpret. In 1993, the prevalence of OSA with greater than or equal to 5 events/hour level in the middle-aged population was reported as 24% for men and 9% for women.[21] For the greater than or equal to 15 events/hour level considered moderate-to-severe disease, a prevalence of 9% and 4% was found. Current studies show a prevalence of up to 23% in women and 50% in men of moderate-to-severe OSA.[22] This increase could equally be explained by increased levels of obesity, by changes in scoring criteria as described earlier, by improved detection sensitivity of sensors, and any combination thereof.[23] For example, using a nasal pressure transducer instead of the older thermistors as the main airflow sensor significantly affects the number of hypopnea events scored, as the thermistor does not detect subtle changes in airflow. Even using the strictest criteria by current AASM standards (hypopneas scored with ≥4% desaturations only), OSA is highly prevalent in society and many subjects are asymptomatic, meaning we do not know whether they benefit from treatment or not.[24] Because the AHI is also used as a diagnostic indicator for whether OSA treatment is successful, this may explain some of the inconclusive results currently being reported related to treatment benefits.[25]

DISCREPANCIES IN THE MEASUREMENTS USED FOR OBSTRUCTIVE SLEEP APNEA SEVERITY

A typical overnight sleep study consists of 8 or more signals. Even with the seemingly clear definitions of an AHI event there are several obstacles to straightforward scoring.

Levels of deoxygenation seem to vary highly between patients with OSA. Patients can experience decreases within normal oxygenation levels (≥90%) or have significant hypoxia, with levels becoming lower than 70% oxygenation. Blood oxygen levels have been used for patient screening for OSA,[26] and deep learning analysis of the pattern of SpO_2 levels has been reported as able to diagnose OSA with significant accuracy.[27] There are important caveats to these results however. Significant variations exist between manufacturers in the SpO_2 values recorded, and it may not be appreciated that readings are heavily preprocessed before analysis to normalize the signal for display.[28,29] SpO_2 sensors are generally not validated for either abnormally low measurements or the rapid changes in oxygenation seen in OSA. The baseline reading has a ±2% accuracy, which complicates comparisons. Obese patients are more likely to have significant hypoxia than lean patients; therefore, screening based solely on SpO_2 levels will likely not be as sensitive in lean patients. There can also be significant variations in individual readings depending on patient skin color and the finger that the sensor is placed

on.[30] Any reliance on absolute measurements in assessment, for example, "SpO_2 measurement less than 90%" or "minimum SpO_2 level" should consequently be treated very carefully, and it should also be considered that abnormally low measurements may not actually be that low.

For the airflow signal measured with a nasal pressure transducer, some manufacturers and sleep laboratories continue to use the older raw pressure signal, which has higher discrepancies in human scoring, instead of a square root transformed flow signal, which has been shown to more closely match the actual airflow in milliliter (Fig. 3).[31] Although some scoring rules require a 30% airflow reduction in order to count hypopneas, others require 50%, using either the raw or the transformed flow signals, giving large variations in scoring, and another instance where older and newer datasets may need to be independently calibrated.

A defining element of an AHI event is that the patient experiences an arousal from sleep, which is typically done from the EEG by detecting a clear transition from a sleeping state. Ideally, arousal scoring would also include an assessment of the sleep stage patients were transitioning from, because the impact on health may differ depending on sleep stage; however, this has yet to be included in the criteria. Correctly labeling the actual sleep stage from EEG readings is problematic. The standard rules that originate from Rechtschaffen and Kales (R&K, 1968)[32] were originally intended to be a reference method, rather than the gold standard for diagnosis that they have become.[33] These rules were used until 2007, when they were replaced by the AASM's scoring manual. Today sleep is categorized as having 2 very distinct states, REM and non-REM, which is now classified as 3 stages of progressive depth (N1, N2, and N3).[34] R&K originally defined 5 sleep stages that were collapsed into 4 by the AASM by combining the older stage 3 and 4 sleep into stage N3 as well as changing some other scoring criteria. Older reference datasets have not typically been rescored against these new guidelines though.

Putting aside the measurement problems in the components of the AHI, there is the problem of the index itself, which measures the frequency of events but not their severity.[35] A long and deep period of breathing cessation is treated the same as a short one, provided it meets the threshold for detection, although the physiologic mechanisms involved suggest that the longer incident is potentially more damaging. If the mechanism for OSA is simply interruption of any of the normal phases of sleep, even one significant incident in

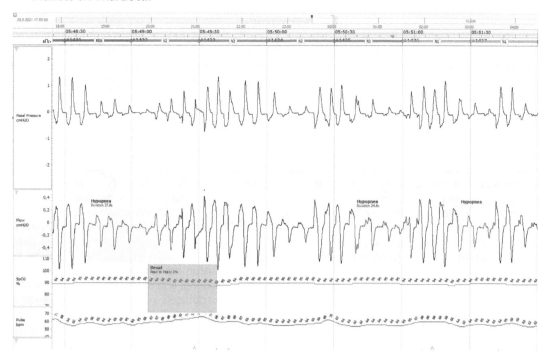

Figure 3. Differences in raw nasal pressure versus transformed nasal flow. The differences in amplitude for the raw signal (*blue line*) are much more pronounced than in the transformed signal (*black line*), which is more highly correlated with milliliter of air. This can have marked effects on the scoring of hypopneas in some patients.

90 minutes could be sufficient to cause problems for the patient, especially if it occurred during REM sleep, but would not be enough to meet diagnostic criteria. Patients with the same absolute AHI score may consequently have very different patterns of OSA severity and symptoms, which can be a confounding factor both in diagnosis and treatment options, as well as attempts to automatically measure AHI.

There is also evidence implicating these issues in the assessment of OSA treatments. A meta-analysis of OSA trials and treatments in 2017 reported uncertainty about the accuracy or clinical utility of different OSA treatments.[25] In particular it has not been established that the standard treatment of OSA using positive airway pressure reduces mortality, or improves other health outcomes, even though it has been shown to reduce the AHI index, subjective sleepiness, and blood pressure scores.

These issues are relatively insignificant for patients with severe OSA but are highly problematic for patients with mild OSA, positional OSA, or REM OSA who may benefit from early intervention but do not have a high enough AHI to be classified as needing treatment. A follow-up of patients with a high probability of OSA based on pretest questionnaire, but who were diagnosed as not having OSA after a home test score of less than 5, showed that 20% had false-negative results on retest.[36] False-positives rates can be equally

problematic especially when screening for OSA is required for employment.[37]

Although the output of the OSA diagnosis process seems to produce clear labels, with well-defined criteria suitable for machine learning, the reality of these measurements can be questioned, with both over- and underdiagnosis being present, and this is dangerous. Machine learning research is often performed by computer specialists who lack an appropriate medical background and also tend to take a mechanical approach to matching human scoring. Equally undue trust is often placed by noncomputer scientists on results with the label of "Artificial Intelligence," when a better description of the techniques involved might be advanced pattern matching. Both medical and machine learning papers that rely on AHI measurements as an absolute ground truth for OSA may be confounded by the scoring criteria itself, rather than the condition. There are also significant statistical issues with assigning hard cutoff and confidence levels to what is potentially a relatively small number of critical events over the course of a night of sleep monitoring.

AUTOMATIC ANALYSIS OF OBSTRUCTIVE SLEEP APNEA

There is a long history of research on automatic analysis of OSA, but efforts have been hindered until recently by a lack of large, easily accessible digitized datasets. Older work was forced to focus mostly on small datasets due to the high cost of conducting sleep studies, making their results at best indicative, because they lack statistical validation. The emergence of HSATs, which allow patients to perform recordings in their own home, has led to a very rapid increase in the size of the available datasets in recent years. Manual scoring of this data is understandably lagging behind.

AASM rules as currently applied to EEG sleep staging represent an interesting trap for any form of statistically based machine analysis that does not carefully consider the expected proportion of time spent in each sleep stage, as this is not evenly distributed across the night. Sleep stage detecting algorithms typically report very different accuracy rates for the different sleep stages, to some extent probabilistically influenced by the distribution of time within the different stages. Equally problematic is that the transition from one stage to another is generally gradual; classification is done by the relative strength of key features; theta waves (4–7 Hz) and sleep spindles are more present in lighter NREM sleep and delta waves (1–4 Hz) in deeper NREM sleep. But features strongly associated with one sleep stage can also be seen in adjacent stages. Human scoring takes this into account and maintains the ordered, "known" transition between sleep stages. Machine learning algorithms without some form of long-term state persistence frequently mislabel segments, and this raises a potential research question as to whether these "misclassifications" by machine learning might include more detailed information about the sleep state then the long states of sleep stage scoring currently being imposed.

Data collection with home recordings encounters the typical issues of an uncontrolled environment. For example, signal input can be noisy, sensors can drop off during sleep, and microphone position can affect the sound recording, as can background noise including partner snoring. Especially in cases of mild sleep apnea, these are all significant confounding issues due to the relatively small number of events required for the AHI. Some of these issues are typically dealt with using filtering and feature preprocessing, but these methods can also vary between researchers and manufacturers, raising further calibration problems.

With the larger datasets now being created, differences in the standards being applied are equally problematic. If algorithms are to be reliably compared, then the version of the scoring standard used to create the algorithm must be reported. But this is not always the case. This is also an issue for manual labeling especially when interrater reliability is being assessed between different specialists.[7] It is suspected these variations may be particularly confounding to deep learning approaches, especially when they use multiple datasets to overcome the relatively small number of labeled datasets available for training. A recent example used separate labeled datasets from Physionet, one recorded in 2013 and the other in 2018.[38] Whether labeling was performed using the same guidelines is not clear from either paper or dataset information, but it seems doubtful.

Machine learning in this area is consequently much more challenging than it may seem. The danger of fitting results to expectations is always present with any form of algorithmic analysis, but it is especially present with deep learning and neural network approaches, which operate on a black box basis, where results that do not conform to the input labeling set will typically be disregarded. It is not hard to find examples. A Convolutional Neural Network architecture trained on a nasal flow cannula sensor to detect OSA reports a Cohen's kappa of 0.81 for severe OSA, but 0.78, 0.71, and 0.69, respectively, for no to moderate OSA. Interestingly, the stated reason in the paper for the reduction in confidence was that the number of AHI events was overestimated by the network. It is equally possible that the network was picking up a valid signal and reacted to events that were missed by manual scoring.[39]

Recent work has pointed to the possibility of improved machine analysis through alternate features, in part by examining whether there was the greatest amount of agreement within human scorers, in this case the SpO_2 desaturation criteria.[40] Because efforts to perform sleep staging from non-EEG signals often throw up issues due to discrepancies between physiologic behavior and sleep stage scoring, especially when patients with OSA are involved: this may also be an area where scoring criteria are proving problematic.[41]

Supporting the idea that OSA is a more complex condition than the current diagnosis criteria allow, evidence has been reported for different phenotypes of the disease in patients with mild OSA. This evidence stems from an examination of the relevant features for classification decisions on individuals in a 48-patient study using DeepLift, a technique for determining the importance of the classifiers in the neural network for the decision.[38,42]

Of considerable concern, if the issues discussed here are not addressed, is the very real possibility that patients with mild OSA, or distinct phenotypes, by virtue of not being classified with the disease, will not be present in the training data used for deep learning approaches and will thus be further excluded from treatment by automatic labeling in the future.

SUMMARY

Both the lack of standardization and the cutoff threshold approach used by the AASM are highly problematic for machine learning attempts to diagnose OSA and other sleep disorders. The typical goal of many machine learning papers is to simplistically match or exceed current human accuracy in scoring. With the uncertainties the authors have described, this is not necessarily a useful goal and may even be a dangerous one. Automatic algorithmic diagnosis can provide a semblance of confidence that is not always well founded. Deep learning approaches can be particularly problematic in this regard, because there is little information on what features the neural networks are actually detecting in the signals, as opposed to the more analytical traditions of signal processing. Deep learning algorithms are often heavily dependent on their input data, so the lack of consistency in scoring and signal calibration can easily create "solutions" that cannot be reproduced on different datasets.

Given the many and various complexities of both the condition and its measurement, the authors recommend that machine learning approaches concentrate on further supporting the development of better diagnostic criteria, and improved understanding of the underlying features of the condition, in partnership with sleep professionals specialized in this area, and this will require large patient and general population datasets with information on symptoms and comorbidities and long-term follow-up. The role of different scoring criteria and other signals of interest such as snoring could then be compared for clinical significance. Although more reliable automatic analysis of sleep studies will reduce the workload of sleep professionals significantly when it is available, it must be reliable. As we continue to rely on manual scoring assisted by automatic analysis, we should include the scorers in the process by reporting the algorithmic confidence levels to the scorer and not just the scores themselves. Exposing this information to scorers would create a channel where feedback could be provided from scorers familiar with the issues in scoring, on any areas that were consistently incorrect due to undue machine confidence, and the same could also be applied in reverse. Human scorers can also be uncertain about labels, analyzing the sources of this uncertainty could provide equally useful insights for improving machine scoring.

Not enough is currently known about patient variability within the condition, in particular with questions on the distribution of OSA events between the different sleep stages, and their impact on the patient's sleep status. Do all patients experience the same pattern of sleep stage response to an event? What impact does the event's severity, measured by duration and deoxygenation, have on their overall and long-term status? Modern instruments provide much more detailed signals, and this information can now be assessed. Night-to-night variability is also indicated as a source of issues with correct diagnosis of moderate sleep apnea, although this may also be another indication of issues with cutoff thresholds.[43] The question of specific patterns to the disease's progression over time, which may affect patient response to treatment, also needs to be judged cautiously with respect to changes in scoring standards.

Treatment of this condition is currently problematic, with the efficacy of the standard treatment using positive air pressure machines being questioned. These machines are also under active development and are starting to automatically analyze the patient condition and attempt to react to it better. Here again considerable care is needed in the application of automated treatment.

Although the development in the last few years of improved machine learning techniques and increasingly large datasets of sleep readings offer considerable opportunity, it is also still in its infancy for OSA. The authors recommend concentrating on basic research and contributing to the creation of a better scoring standard and avoiding attempts to merely replicate current human scoring. The large datasets that are beginning to be available present considerable opportunities in terms of analyzing the different ways the disease can present, its detection, and if included in longitudinal studies, how it develops, and the effects of treatment. In time this work can lead to far better diagnostic criteria than the current AHI.

CLINICS CARE POINTS

- When performing novel machine learning analyses on sleep data, it is highly recommended to work interdisciplinarily with relevant sleep specialists.
- When using manual sleep study scoring for machine learning purposes, be aware of the different scoring standards available and scoring uncertainties.

- Do not consider existing diagnostic and measurement criteria as a gold standard that cannot be changed—validation of new, improved criteria is needed in many cases.
- Do assess critically the signals used that will be used in machine learning, to understand their limitations moving forward in the work.
- Reliable, automatic analysis of sleep data is sorely needed for the different signals assessed in sleep studies.

DISCLOSURE

No relevant conflict of interest to disclose.

REFERENCE

1. Redline S, Dean D, Sanders MH. Entering the Era of "Big data": getting our metrics right. Sleep 2013; 36(4):465–9.
2. Marcus CL. Obstructive sleep apnea syndrome: differences between children and adults. Sleep 2000; 23(Suppl 4):S140–1.
3. Arnardottir ES, Mackiewicz M, Gislason T, et al. Molecular signatures of obstructive sleep apnea in adults: a review and perspective. Sleep 2009;32(4):447–70.
4. Berry RB, Brooks R, Gamaldo CE, et al. The AASM manual for the scoring of sleep and associated events; rules, terminology and technical specifications. American Academy of Sleep Medicine; 2015 Version 2.2. .
5. Kapur VK, Auckley DH, Chowdhuri S, et al. Clinical practice guideline for diagnostic testing for adult obstructive sleep apnea: an American Academy of sleep medicine clinical practice guideline. J Clin Sleep Med 2017;13(03):479–504.
6. Miettinen T, Myllymaa K, Westeren-Punnonen S, et al. Success rate and technical quality of home polysomnography with self-applicable electrode set in subjects with possible sleep Bruxism. IEEE J Biomed Health Inform 2018;22(4):1124–32.
7. Deng S, Zhang X, Zhang Y, et al. Interrater agreement between American and Chinese sleep centers according to the 2014 AASM standard. Sleep Breath 2019;23(2):719–28.
8. Benjafield A, Valentine K, Ayas N, et al. Global prevalence of obstructive sleep apnea in adults: estimation using currently available data. In: B67. Risk and prevalence OF sleep DISORDERED breathing. American Thoracic society International Conference Abstracts. American Thoracic Society; 2018. p. A3962. https://doi.org/10.1164/ajrccm-conference. 2018.197.1_MeetingAbstracts.A3962.
9. Sleep-related breathing disorders in adults: recommendations for syndrome definition and measurement techniques in clinical research. The Report of an American Academy of Sleep Medicine Task Force. Sleep 1999;22(5):667–89.
10. Kuna ST, Benca R, Kushida CA, et al. Agreement in computer-assisted manual scoring of Polysomnograms across sleep centers. Sleep 2013;36(4): 583–9.
11. Hirotsu C, Haba-Rubio J, Andries D, et al. Effect of three hypopnea scoring criteria on OSA prevalence and associated comorbidities in the general population. J Clin Sleep Med 2019;15(2):183–94.
12. Pevernagie DA, Gnidovec-Strazisar B, Grote L, et al. On the rise and fall of the apnea–hypopnea index: a historical review and critical appraisal. J Sleep Res 2020;29(4):e13066.
13. Arnardottir ES, Gislason T. Quantifying airflow limitation and snoring during sleep. Sleep Med Clin 2016; 11(4):421–34.
14. Alzoubaidi M, Mokhlesi B. Obstructive sleep apnea during rapid eye movement sleep: clinical relevance and therapeutic implications. Curr Opin Pulm Med 2016;22(6):545–54.
15. Garvey JF, Pengo MF, Drakatos P, et al. Epidemiological aspects of obstructive sleep apnea. J Thorac Dis 2015;7(5):920–9.
16. Ryan S, Crinion SJ, McNicholas WT. Obesity and sleep-disordered breathing–when two "bad guys" meet. QJM 2014;107(12):949–54.
17. Leinum CJ, Dopp JM, Morgan BJ. Sleep-disordered breathing and obesity: pathophysiology, complications, and treatment. Nutr Clin Pract 2009;24(6): 675–87.
18. Lee SA, Amis TC, Byth K, et al. Heavy snoring as a cause of carotid artery atherosclerosis. Sleep 2008; 31(9):1207–13.
19. Fedson AC, Pack AI, Gislason T. Frequently used sleep questionnaires in epidemiological and genetic research for obstructive sleep apnea: a review. Sleep Med Rev 2012;16(6):529–37.
20. Pataka A, Bonsignore MR, Ryan S, et al. Cancer prevalence is increased in females with sleep apnoea: data from the ESADA study. Eur Respir J 2019;53(6):1900091.
21. Young T, Palta M, Dempsey J, et al. The occurrence of sleep-disordered breathing among middle-aged adults. N Engl J Med 1993;328(17):1230–5.
22. Heinzer R, Vat S, Marques-Vidal P, et al. Prevalence of sleep-disordered breathing in the general population: the HypnoLaus study. Lancet Respir Med 2015; 3(4):310–8.
23. O'Driscoll DM, Landry SA, Pham J, et al. The physiological phenotype of obstructive sleep apnea differs between Caucasian and Chinese patients. Sleep 2019;42(11):zsz186.
24. Arnardottir ES, Bjornsdottir E, Olafsdottir KA, et al. Obstructive sleep apnoea in the general population: highly prevalent but minimal symptoms. Eur Respir J 2016;47(1):194–202.

25. Jonas DE, Amick HR, Feltner C, et al. Screening for obstructive sleep apnea in adults: evidence report and systematic review for the US Preventive Services Task Force. JAMA 2017;317(4):415–33.

26. Ng ASL, Wong TKS, Gohel MDI, et al. Using pulse oximetry level to indicate the occurrence of sleep apnoea events. Stud Health Technol Inform 2006; 122:672–5.

27. Nikkonen S, Afara IO, Leppänen T, et al. Artificial neural network analysis of the oxygen saturation signal enables accurate diagnostics of sleep apnea. Sci Rep 2019;9(1):13200.

28. Xu L, Han F, Keenan BT, et al. Validation of the Nox-T3 portable monitor for diagnosis of obstructive sleep apnea in Chinese adults. J Clin Sleep Med 2017;13(5):675–83.

29. Chang Y, Xu L, Han F, et al. Validation of the Nox-T3 portable monitor for diagnosis of obstructive sleep apnea in patients with Chronic obstructive Pulmonary disease. J Clin Sleep Med 2019;15(4):587–96.

30. Basaranoglu G, Bakan M, Umutoglu T, et al. Comparison of SpO2 values from different fingers of the hands. SpringerPlus 2015;4(1):561.

31. Farré R, Rigau J, Montserrat JM, et al. Relevance of linearizing nasal prongs for assessing hypopneas and flow limitation during sleep. Am J Respir Crit Care Med 2001;163(2):494–7.

32. Wolpert EA. A manual of standardized terminology, techniques and scoring system for sleep stages of human subjects. Arch Gen Psychiatry 1969;20(2): 246.

33. Himanen S-L, Hasan J. Limitations of rechtschaffen and kales. Sleep Med Rev 2000;4(2):149–67.

34. Silber MH, Ancoli-Israel S, Bonnet MH, et al. The visual scoring of sleep in adults. J Clin Sleep Med 2007;3(2):121–31.

35. Borsini E, Nogueira F, Nigro C. Apnea-hypopnea index in sleep studies and the risk of over-simplification. Sleep Sci 2018;11(1):45–8.

36. Stanchina MI, Prenda S, Lincoln J, et al. Negative home sleep testing in patients with high risk obstructive sleep apnea Characteristics. In: B66. SRN: Current and emerging treatment therapies to improve sleep. American Thoracic society international Conference Abstracts. Am Thorac Soc 2019;A3908. https://doi.org/10.1164/ajrccm-conference.2019.199.1_MeetingAbstracts.A3908.

37. Berger M, Varvarigou V, Rielly A, et al. Employer-mandated sleep apnea screening and diagnosis in commercial drivers. J Occup Environ Med 2012; 54(8):1017–25.

38. Mousavi S, Afghah F, Acharya UR. SleepEEGNet: automated sleep stage scoring with sequence to sequence deep learning approach. PLOS ONE 2019;14(5):e0216456.

39. Choi SH, Yoon H, Kim HS, et al. Real-time apnea-hypopnea event detection during sleep by convolutional neural networks. Comput Biol Med 2018;100: 123–31.

40. Biswal S, Sun H, Goparaju B, et al. Expert-level sleep scoring with deep neural networks. J Am Med Inform Assoc 2018;25(12):1643–50.

41. Sun H, Ganglberger W, Panneerselvam E, et al. Sleep staging from electrocardiography and respiration with deep learning. Sleep 2019;21. https://doi.org/10.1093/sleep/zsz306. zsz306.

42. Jansen C, Hodel S, Penzel T, et al. Feature relevance in physiological networks for classification of obstructive sleep apnea. Physiol Meas 2018; 39(12):124003.

43. Stöberl AS, Schwarz EI, Haile SR, et al. Night-to-night variability of obstructive sleep apnea. J Sleep Res 2017;26(6):782–8.

Getting More from the Sleep Recording

Walter T. McNicholas, MD, FERS

KEYWORDS

- Obstructive sleep apnea • Signal processing • Oximetry • Acoustic recording • Pulse transit time
- Actigraphy • Biosensors

KEY POINTS

- Developments in signal processing facilitate the automated analysis of traditional signals such as oxygen saturation and electroencephalogram, which provides superior insight into physiology and pathophysiology compared to manual analysis.
- These developments have resulted in increasing recognition that the traditional measure of sleep-disordered breathing, the apnea-hypopnea index, is a poor predictor of disease significance.
- New approaches to the recording and analysis of traditional signals such as snoring and oxygen saturation facilitate ambulatory diagnosis of obstructive sleep apnea.
- Detailed insight into the characteristics of oxygen desaturation during sleep provides superior prediction of comorbidities than the apnea-hypopnea index.
- Derivatives of the electrocardiogram and pulse wave provide indirect data on sleep-disordered breathing that are suitable for ambulatory diagnosis.

INTRODUCTION

Sleep recordings have been a feature of clinical sleep practice for more than 4 decades, and full sleep laboratory recordings in the form of polysomnography (PSG) remain largely based on principles established in these early years. Sleep staging remains fundamentally based on the scoring rules established by Rechtschaffen and Kales in 1968,[1] and the scoring of sleep-disordered breathing (SDB) events is based on the so-called Chicago Criteria introduced in 1999, which also proposed a severity grading for obstructive sleep apnea (OSA) based on the frequency of apneas and hypopneas per hour of sleep (AHI).[2] However, developments in technology and signal analysis in more recent years offer considerable scope to expand and enhance the information that can be obtained from sleep studies, and advances in the understanding of mechanisms contributing to cardiometabolic comorbidities offer new insights regarding the most important sleep-related variables that contribute

to these comorbidities.[3] There has been increasing interest among the sleep research community in exploring new and novel approaches to the diagnosis of sleep disorders, especially OSA, and there is increasing recognition that variables such as the AHI may not be the most important measure to quantify the severity of the disorder.[4]

The focus of this review is to explore how additional information may be obtained from signals obtained in traditional sleep recordings such as laboratory-based PSG and home-based sleep studies, as well as information from additional signals that do not form part of traditional sleep studies. The review will focus primarily on the assessment of patients with suspected OSA, as the high prevalence of this disorder, which affects up to one billion subjects worldwide,[5] makes it particularly relevant to explore novel approaches to the accurate and reliable diagnosis of this disorder in the ambulatory setting.[6]

Currently, disease severity is measured using AHI as determined from a sleep study. However, there is poor association between daytime

Department of Respiratory and Sleep Medicine, School of Medicine, University College Dublin, St. Vincent's Hospital Group, Elm Park, Dublin 4, Ireland
E-mail address: walter.mcnicholas@ucd.ie

Sleep Med Clin 16 (2021) 567–574
https://doi.org/10.1016/j.jsmc.2021.08.001
1556-407X/21/© 2021 The Author(s). Published by Elsevier Inc. This is an open access article under the CC BY license (http://creativecommons.org/licenses/by/4.0/).

symptoms such as excessive daytime sleepiness and the AHI,[7] and there is increasing evidence that cardiometabolic comorbidities may be more related to measures of oxygen desaturation during sleep than the AHI.[3] Thus, there is increasing interest in moving away from the AHI as the most important measure of OSA severity toward a more personalized approach to OSA diagnosis and treatment,[8] which considers individual risk factors, clinical history, and comorbid disease in the diagnosis and treatment of each patient with OSA.

INDIVIDUAL PATIENT PHENOTYPING

While overnight diagnostic sleep studies provide the core evidence of SDB in patients with suspected OSA, there is clear evidence that the sleep study alone does not provide sufficient evidence for the diagnosis of the clinical syndrome. This aspect has been recognized for many years,[9,10] and more recently, there is strong evidence that clusters of different clinical phenotypes can be identified among the broad population of patients presenting for assessment.[11] Furthermore, certain pathophysiological traits that are very common in OSA such as loss of nocturnal dipping of blood pressure (BP) have significant implications for the development of associated comorbidity.[12] Thus, whatever sleep study is used in the assessment of suspected OSA, the findings must be integrated into the overall assessment of the patient as regards clinical significance, and management should be linked to the underlying clinical and pathophysiological phenotypes where additional factors to the AHI such as acute systemic effects and associated relevant comorbidity are factored into the decision-making process.[8] A further consideration in the clinical assessment of OSA is the role of the AHI alone, referred to here in this context as SDB. Although the International Classification of Sleep Disorders refers to AHI $\geq$ 15 as sufficient for a diagnosis of OSA, this appears questionable in the context of this level of SDB being reported in up to 50% of a normal adult male population.[13]

DEVELOPMENTS IN THE ANALYSIS OF EXISTING SIGNALS

Core signals relevant to sleep and breathing disorders such as airflow, oxygen saturation, and cardiac variables have been included in sleep studies for decades, but developments in signal analysis have permitted enhanced and clinically relevant information to be obtained, which significantly adds to the diagnostic potential of the studies concerned. Furthermore, novel approaches to the analysis of these traditional signals may facilitate the use of limited diagnostic systems that may be especially useful in the ambulatory setting.

ELECTROENCEPHALOGRAPHY AND SLEEP STAGING

Developments in electroencephalographic (EEG) recording technology have permitted the introduction of ambulatory EEG recordings, which may use a full EEG montage. This technology is not necessary in most clinical situations involved in the assessment of OSA, although some limited ear-based EEG recording systems have been developed that are easy to apply and may provide additional useful information in the ambulatory respiratory-sleep clinical setting.[14]

Specialized computer-based analysis of the EEG by techniques such as spectral analysis provides additional insight into sleep physiology and pathology beyond traditional sleep staging, but these are research-oriented and have little application in the clinical setting of respiratory sleep disorders.[15,16]

ACOUSTIC AND AIRFLOW DEVICES
Acoustic Devices

Although snoring is a common feature in patients with OSA, the symptom has limited value on its own in the assessment of OSA because of its weak relationship with the AHI.[17] Nonetheless, the detailed characteristics of snoring and, especially, the characteristic intermittent nature of snoring in patients with OSA provide potential diagnostic utility both alone and in combination with other signals. In this context, periods of apnea/hypopnea have quite different acoustic characteristics to nonapneic snoring. One such acoustic device is BresoDX (BresoTEC Inc, Toronto, Ontario, Canada), which is a portable device that consists of a lightweight face frame, which contains an embedded electronic module and microphone. Recorded sounds are continually stored and can subsequently be downloaded for analysis.[18,19] As might be expected, a characteristic cyclical intermittent pattern of snoring has the greatest predictive potential for the diagnosis of OSA. In one report of 135 subjects with suspected OSA, the calculated AHI using BresoDX showed a relatively good correlation with PSG and demonstrated a diagnostic accuracy ranging between 88.9% and 93.3% at AHI cutoffs of 5 to 15.[20] More recently, an over the counter small, wireless wearable patch has been developed

(Zansors, Arlington, VA), which estimates breathing patterns using an inbuilt microphone and includes an accelerometer to record movement. A pilot study of the device demonstrated 75% sensitivity and 71% specificity for detecting SDB compared to gold standard PSG.[21]

Airflow Devices

Devices that record airflow by nasal pressure recordings as a single measure have been developed as a more simple ambulatory diagnostic technique for OSA, and an example of such a device is the ApneaLink (Resmed, Sydney, Australia).[22] One report comparing the device with PSG showed a 73.1% sensitivity and 91% specificity for detecting an AHI greater than 15 in at-risk populations,[23] with similar results reported in other studies.[22,24]

OXIMETRY

Overnight oximetry has long been proposed as a simple and reasonably accurate technique for OSA diagnosis, especially in severe cases,[10,25] but has limited reliability in mild OSA where oxygen desaturations may be relatively minor. To be useful in the assessment of patients with OSA, arterial oxygen saturation (SpO2) recordings require a high sampling rate (>0.5 Hz) to ensure detection of the intermittent oxygen desaturations that are characteristic of the disorder. In clinical practice, several relevant variables may be obtained from the recordings, including the oxygen desaturation index (ODI), which is the number of desaturations per hour which drop ≥3% (ODI3) or ≥4% (ODI4) below the baseline level, and the cumulative time with an SpO2 below a predetermined level, usually 90% (T90). Additional information can be obtained from the SpO2 variability, referred to as the delta index.[26,27] In OSA, a "saw-tooth" pattern of recurring transient oxygen desaturations is seen, especially in severe cases, which provides a unique visual picture of the disorder. Simple indices such as the ODI may fail to capture all the important and potentially relevant pathophysiological characteristics[25] and novel strategies for the analysis of oximetry using automated techniques[28–30] to help maximize the diagnostic potential of SpO2 data. Furthermore, novel approaches to oxygen desaturation such as the hypoxic burden have been demonstrated to provide a superior prediction of cardiovascular morbidity and mortality than the AHI in large-population studies.[31]

Computer-assisted applications that provide automated signal processing facilitate the quantification of the frequency, duration, and severity of desaturations, which enhance the clinical assessment of OSA.[29,32–34] Some devices use smartphone-based technology or wearable applications as the receiver which may have potential for home screening to prioritize cases for more detailed investigation[35–37] and may also have a role in treatment follow-up.[38]

Oximetry and Apneas and Hypopneas per Hour of Sleep

The ODI may be used as an alternative to the AHI to quantify the number of respiratory events during the night but may underestimate the severity of OSA with potentially important clinical consequences[39,40] that may influence treatment decisions.[26] However, a more detailed analysis of the SpO2 signal with computer-assisted and machine learning algorithms improves the predictive ability[41–43] with a diagnostic accuracy of up to 96.7% reported. Furthermore, there is growing evidence that measures of oxygen desaturation are superior to AHI in the prediction of comorbidities including hypertension (HTN),[44] diabetes mellitus,[45] and heart failure.[46]

Oximetry may also have value in screening patients for OSA in certain comorbidities including stroke,[47] heart failure,[48] morbid obesity,[49,50] and chronic obstructive pulmonary disease (COPD).[51] In stroke, OSA is associated with diminished recovery and increased mortality.[52] In patients with congestive cardiac failure, overnight oximetry has a high sensitivity (97%) but poor specificity (32%) for SDB.[48] Oximetry performs better in patients with gross obesity with reports of up to 100% sensitivity and 93% specificity for SDB in ambulatory testing.[49] Oximetry has limited potential for the diagnosis of OSA in patients with COPD with low sensitivity (59%) and specificity (60%)[51] although performs better when combined with novel signal analysis technology.[53]

Cardiac Based Measures

Electrocardiograph (ECG) analysis: monitoring of heart rate variability (HRV), electrocardiograph morphology, and respiration

Monitoring of HRV by overnight ECG has long been recognized as a potential diagnostic tool in patients with SDB.[54] In standard PSG, a single-lead ECG is recorded to allow measurement of heart rate and rhythm. A special dedicated software program allows analysis of HRV[55] that can provide information relating to autonomic activity and may give added insight into sleep stages.[56] Further information can be obtained from fluctuations in the QRS amplitude that are a consequence of rib cage movements during respiration. The combination of ECG-derived respiratory movement and sleep apnea–related HRV has the potential to be a useful screening tool for OSA[57] and has the added value of being available in a typical cardiology setting, which provides the potential for screening in this setting before referral to a sleep clinic.

Pulse transit time

The pulse transit time (PTT) is a variable that is derived from the ECG and the arterial pressure wave measured by a finger probe and has been reported to reflect inspiratory effort.[58] PTT measures the time taken for the arterial pulse wave to travel between the aortic valve (R wave on ECG) and the finger blood vessels as indicated by pulse oximetry. Pulse wave speed varies with arterial stiffness, which in turn is influenced by the BP level. PTT has been reported to give an indirect measure of both apnea and arousal.[58]

Peripheral arterial tonometry (the pulse wave as a measure)

Peripheral arterial tonometry (PAT) provides a detailed assessment of the pulse wave and is reported to be a relatively robust diagnostic screening method for OSA. The pulse wave amplitude is influenced by sympathetic tone, and arousals are also associated with a drop in pulse amplitude. Furthermore, the pulse rate also provides an indirect assessment of sleep stage.[59] WatchPAT (Itamar Medical, Caesarea, Israel) uses a proprietary algorithm combining PAT data, oxygen saturation, pulse rate, and actigraphy that generates an estimate of total sleep time and calculates an AHI.[60] WatchPAT has been evaluated in several studies with some, but not all, reports indicating the device to provide a reasonably accurate assessment of OSA.[59–61] A meta-analysis found a good correlation between sleep indices calculated by laboratory-based PSG and those obtained from a PAT device (r = 0.889),[62] thus supporting its use as a viable ambulatory diagnostic tool for OSA.

Blood pressure monitoring as a potential diagnostic tool

OSA is a recognized independent risk factor for systemic HTN, and obstructive apneas may lead to acute BP elevation during sleep,[12,63] which can result in a loss of the normal nocturnal dipping pattern of BP. A recent meta-analysis found that OSA is associated with a 1.5-fold increase in the prevalence of nondipping BP,[64] thus suggesting that ambulatory BP monitoring (ABPM) could serve as a surrogate marker for OSA. Support for this possibility comes from reports that nondipping nocturnal BP predicts OSA in subjects undergoing

ABPM.[65] Furthermore, a recent report from this department indicated a high predictive value for moderate to severe OSA in unselected patients recruited from a HTN clinic who had a nondipping pattern of nocturnal BP on 24-hour ABPM.[66] These findings support the possibility that ABPM may be a useful biomarker for OSA, irrespective of the clinical index of suspicion for the disorder.

Limitations of ABPM with a pneumatic cuff include the possibility that cuff inflation causes arousal and that the device is unable to track rapid changes in BP associated with individual apneas.[67,68] Such limitations may be overcome by continuous measurement of BP by finger photoplethysmography, which uses a small cuff fitted to the finger that provides a continuous measurement. This device provides beat-by-beat pressure measurements and gives an indication of BP variability, which is typically increased in OSA.[69] A novel smart-watch, CareUp (Farasha Labs, Paris, France), has been developed that gives a continuous estimation of BP[70] and has been validated in a study of 44 subjects.[67] This simple device may provide an additional method for home BP monitoring, which could be a promising screening method for OSA, although further research of this technique is required before being accepted into clinical practice.

ACTIGRAPHY

Sleep is associated with reduced body motion compared to wakefulness, and lack of body movement is widely used as a surrogate marker for sleep. Actigraphy is the most widely used method, and typically uses an accelerometer that is either a stand-alone device or built into a wristwatch. Actigraphy can be used to estimate daily sleep-wake cycles, which can be clinically useful in the evaluation of many sleep disorders. Actigraphy has been formally evaluated by the American Academy of Sleep Medicine and recognized as a valid research tool in sleep[71] and, more recently, as an alternative to PSG for prolonged monitoring of sleep quality.[72] Several reviews[73–75] have indicated that actigraphy can provide clinically useful information about sleep in the natural environment, which may assist in clinical decision-making. However, actigraphy is not reliable in distinguishing different sleep stages and has poor specificity.[76] In comparison with PSG, actigraphy overestimates total sleep time and underestimates time spent awake.[77] Actigraphy provides an indirect signal relating to body motion, which implies that estimation of sleep stages is only derived from an assessment of how body motion changes during different sleep stages, and is likely

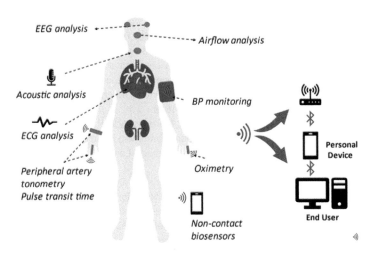

Fig. 1. Potential physiologic signals for the diagnosis and monitoring of OSA. Signals can be fed wirelessly or via Bluetooth to a router or smartphone and then uploaded to a secured database, whereby end users may access and review the data. BP, blood pressure; ECG, electrocardiogram; EEG, electroencephalogram.

to be of limited accuracy in this determination. However, with improving technology, the role of actigraphy as a screening tool will likely increase and be included in ambulatory diagnostic systems for OSA where accurate measures of sleep staging are not generally required.

Wireless Systems – Biosensors in Obstructive Sleep Apnea

Wireless monitoring systems have been in clinical use for several decades, and an early example involved pressure-sensitive foils placed over the mattress, which provided measures of sleep, heart rate, and respiration.[78] Wireless devices have greatly improved over subsequent years and benefit from developments in digital technology that are used in signal acquisition and processing.

Radio frequency waves, which are similar to radar technology, can detect small body movements, such as those produced by respiration, which may facilitate the assessment of sleep and wakefulness and of SDB. SleepMinder (ResMed Sensor Technologies, Dublin, Ireland) is a noncontact device that estimates the severity of SDB using a multichannel biomotion sensor and an integrated analysis software program.[79] The device has been shown to correlate well with PSG in the determination of AHI[80] and sleep efficiency[81] during controlled laboratory settings. More recently, the device has been reported to be a useful screening tool in the detection of moderate and severe OSA, although having poor accuracy in the setting of mild OSA.[82]

Actigraphy has been incorporated into many smartphone applications that estimate sleep quality, and additional signals relevant to the assessment of SDB may be obtained from audio and oximetry recordings that have been incorporated into many wearable recording systems, which may also include monitoring of heart rate.[83] Given their wide availability, relatively low cost, and ease of use, smartphones and wearable devices may provide a valuable screening opportunity for the detection of OSA and other sleep disorders,[84,85] which may also help prioritize patients that require more detailed investigation. Finally, technological advances in telemedicine may strengthen interdepartmental collaboration to improve the overall care of OSA patients.[86]

SUMMARY

Developments in signal technology and analysis provide novel approaches to the assessment of patients suspected of OSA, which range from enhanced analysis of traditional signals to novel signal technologies that provide surrogate markers of OSA. The potential range of novel approaches to the assessment of OSA is illustrated in **Fig. 1.**

CLINICS CARE POINTS

- When examining the oximetry tracing for features consistent with OSA, ensure that the technology of the recording device has a sufficiently high sampling rate to detect the characteristic fluctuations in oxygen saturation.

- While snoring does not directly relate to OSA, short gaps during prolonged periods of snoring provide an indirect indication of upper airway obstruction.

> • The absence of nocturnal dipping of blood pressure is a potential surrogate marker of OSA and is especially important as this represents a cardiovascular comorbidity.

DISCLOSURE

The author has nothing to disclose.

REFERENCES

1. Rechtschaffen A, Kales A. A manual of standardized terminology, techniques and scoring system for sleep stages of human subjects. Washington, DC: US Government Printing Office, Public Health Service; 1968.

2. Flemons WW, Buysse D, Redline S, et al. Sleep-related breathing disorders in adults: recommendations for syndrome definition and measurement techniques in clinical research. Sleep 1999;22(5): 667–89.

3. McNicholas WT. Obstructive sleep apnoea and comorbidity - an overview of the association and impact of continuous positive airway pressure therapy. Expert Rev Respir Med 2019;13(3):251–61.

4. Pevernagie DA, Gnidovec-Strazisar B, Grote L, et al. On the rise and fall of the apnea-hypopnea index: a historical review and critical appraisal. J Sleep Res 2020;29(4):e13066.

5. Benjafield AV, Ayas NT, Eastwood PR, et al. Estimation of the global prevalence and burden of obstructive sleep apnoea: a literature-based analysis. Lancet Respir Med 2019;7(8):687–98.

6. O'Mahony AM, Garvey JF, McNicholas WT. Technologic advances in the assessment and management of obstructive sleep apnoea beyond the apnoea-hypopnoea index: a narrative review. J Thorac Dis 2020;12(9):5020–38.

7. Deegan PC, McNicholas WT. Predictive value of clinical features for the obstructive sleep apnoea syndrome. Eur Respir J 1996;9(1):117–24.

8. Randerath W, Bassetti CL, Bonsignore MR, et al. Challenges and perspectives in obstructive sleep apnoea: report by an ad hoc working group of the sleep disordered breathing group of the European respiratory society and the European sleep research society. Eur Respir J 2018;52(3):1702616.

9. Young T, Palta M, Dempsey J, et al. The occurrence of sleep-disordered breathing among middle-aged adults. N Engl J Med 1993;328(17):1230–5.

10. McNicholas WT. Diagnosis of obstructive sleep apnea in adults. Proc Am Thorac Soc 2008;5(2): 154–60.

11. Bailly S, Grote L, Hedner J, et al. Clusters of sleep apnoea phenotypes: a large pan-European study from the European Sleep Apnoea Database (ESADA). Respirology 2021;26(4):378–87.

12. Crinion SJ, Ryan S, McNicholas WT. Obstructive sleep apnoea as a cause of nocturnal nondipping blood pressure: recent evidence regarding clinical importance and underlying mechanisms. Eur Respir J 2017;49(1):1601818.

13. Heinzer R, Vat S, Marques-Vidal P, et al. Prevalence of sleep-disordered breathing in the general population: the HypnoLaus study. Lancet Respir Med 2015; 3(4):310–8.

14. Bleichner MG, Debener S. Concealed, unobtrusive ear-centered EEG acquisition: cEEGrids for transparent EEG. Front Hum Neurosci 2017;11:163.

15. Liu S, Shen J, Li Y, et al. EEG power spectral analysis of abnormal cortical activations during REM/NREM sleep in obstructive sleep apnea. Front Neurol 2021;12:643855.

16. Mainieri G, Maranci J-B, Champetier P, et al. Are sleep paralysis and false awakenings different from REM sleep and from lucid REM sleep? A spectral EEG analysis. J Clin Sleep Med 2021;17(4): 719–27.

17. Alshaer H, Hummel R, Mendelson M, et al. Objective relationship between sleep apnea and frequency of snoring assessed by machine learning. J Clin Sleep Med 2019;15(3):463–70.

18. Alshaer H, Fernie GR, Maki E, et al. Validation of an automated algorithm for detecting apneas and hypopneas by acoustic analysis of breath sounds. Sleep Med 2013;14(6):562–71.

19. Alshaer H, Levchenko A, Bradley TD, et al. A system for portable sleep apnea diagnosis using an embedded data capturing module. J Clin Monit Comput 2013;27(3):303–11.

20. Alshaer H, Fernie GR, Tseng WH, et al. Comparison of in-laboratory and home diagnosis of sleep apnea using a cordless portable acoustic device. Sleep Med 2016;22:91–6.

21. Abbasi J. In-home, over-the-counter sleep apnea sensor on the Horizon. JAMA 2017;317(22):2271.

22. Erman MK, Stewart D, Einhorn D, et al. Validation of the ApneaLink for the screening of sleep apnea: a novel and simple single-channel recording device. J Clin Sleep Med 2007;3(4):387–92.

23. Masa JF, Duran-Cantolla J, Capote F, et al. Effectiveness of home single-channel nasal pressure for sleep apnea diagnosis. Sleep 2014;37(12):1953–61.

24. Oktay B, Rice TB, Atwood CW Jr, et al. Evaluation of a single-channel portable monitor for the diagnosis of obstructive sleep apnea. J Clin Sleep Med 2011;7(4):384–90.

25. Netzer N, Eliasson AH, Netzer C, et al. Overnight pulse oximetry for sleep-disordered breathing in adults: a review. Chest 2001;120(2):625–33.

26. Kapur VK, Auckley DH, Chowdhuri S, et al. Clinical practice guideline for diagnostic testing for adult

obstructive sleep apnea: an American Academy of sleep medicine clinical practice guideline. J Clin Sleep Med 2017;13(3):479–504.

27. Berry RB, Budhiraja R, Gottlieb DJ, et al. Rules for scoring respiratory events in sleep: update of the 2007 AASM manual for the scoring of sleep and associated events. Deliberations of the sleep apnea definitions task force of the American academy of sleep medicine. J Clin Sleep Med 2012;8(5):597–619.

28. Uddin MB, Chow CM, Su SW. Classification methods to detect sleep apnea in adults based on respiratory and oximetry signals: a systematic review. Physiol Meas 2018;39(3):03TR01.

29. Del Campo F, Crespo A, Cerezo-Hernandez A, et al. Oximetry use in obstructive sleep apnea. Expert Rev Respir Med 2018;12(8):665–81.

30. Mendonca F, Mostafa SS, Ravelo-Garcia AG, et al. A review of obstructive sleep apnea detection approaches. IEEE J Biomed Health Inform 2019; 23(2):825–37.

31. Azarbarzin A, Sands SA, Stone KL, et al. The hypoxic burden of sleep apnoea predicts cardiovascular disease-related mortality: the osteoporotic fractures in men study and the sleep heart health study. Eur Heart J 2019;40(14):1149–57.

32. Mendonca F, Mostafa SS, Ravelo-Garcia AG, et al. Devices for home detection of obstructive sleep apnea: a review. Sleep Med Rev 2018;41:149–60.

33. Terrill PI. A review of approaches for analysing obstructive sleep apnoea-related patterns in pulse oximetry data. Respirology 2020;25(5): 475–85.

34. Deviaene M, Testelmans D, Buyse B, et al. Automatic screening of sleep apnea patients based on the SpO2 signal. IEEE J Biomed Health Inform 2019;23(2):607–17.

35. Burgos A, Goni A, Illarramendi A, et al. Real-time detection of apneas on a PDA. IEEE Trans Inf Technol Biomed 2010;14(4):995–1002.

36. Zhang J, Zhang Q, Wang Y, et al. A real-time auto-adjustable smart pillow system for sleep apnea detection and treatment. Proceedings of the 12th International conference on Information processing in sensor networks; Philadelphia, Pennsylvania: Association for Computing Machinery. 2013. p. 179–90.

37. Angius G, Raffo L, editors. A sleep apnea keeper in a wearable device for continuous detection and screening during daily life. 2008. Piscataway: IEEE - Institute of Electrical and Electronics Engineers; 2008. p. 433–6.

38. Mendonca F, Mostafa SS, Morgado-Dias F, et al. An oximetry based wireless device for sleep apnea detection. Sensors (Basel) 2020;20(3):888.

39. McNicholas WT, Bonsigore MR. Sleep apnoea as an independent risk factor for cardiovascular disease: current evidence, basic mechanisms and research priorities. Eur Respir J 2007;29(1):156–78.

40. Lam JC, Mak JC, Ip MS. Obesity, obstructive sleep apnoea and metabolic syndrome. Respirology 2012;17(2):223–36.

41. Ebben MR, Krieger AC. Diagnostic accuracy of a mathematical model to predict apnea-hypopnea index using nighttime pulse oximetry. J Biomed Opt 2016;21(3):35006.

42. Jung DW, Hwang SH, Cho JG, et al. Real-time automatic apneic event detection using nocturnal pulse oximetry. IEEE Trans Biomed Eng 2018;65(3):706–12.

43. Marcos JV, Hornero R, Alvarez D, et al. Automated prediction of the apnea-hypopnea index from nocturnal oximetry recordings. IEEE Trans Biomed Eng 2012;59(1):141–9.

44. Tkacova R, McNicholas WT, Javorsky M, et al. Nocturnal intermittent hypoxia predicts prevalent hypertension in the European Sleep Apnoea Database cohort study. Eur Respir J 2014;44(4):931–41.

45. Kent BD, Grote L, Bonsignore MR, et al. Sleep apnoea severity independently predicts glycaemic health in nondiabetic subjects: the ESADA study. Eur Respir J 2014;44(1):130–9.

46. Azarbarzin A, Sands SA, Taranto-Montemurro L, et al. The sleep apnea-specific hypoxic burden predicts Incident heart failure. Chest 2020;158(2):739–50.

47. Aaronson JA, van Bezeij T, van den Aardweg JG, et al. Diagnostic accuracy of nocturnal oximetry for detection of sleep apnea syndrome in stroke rehabilitation. Stroke 2012;43(9):2491–3.

48. Ward NR, Cowie MR, Rosen SD, et al. Utility of overnight pulse oximetry and heart rate variability analysis to screen for sleep-disordered breathing in chronic heart failure. Thorax 2012;67(11):1000–5.

49. Malbois M, Giusti V, Suter M, et al. Oximetry alone versus portable polygraphy for sleep apnea screening before bariatric surgery. Obes Surg 2010;20(3):326–31.

50. Chung F, Liao P, Elsaid H, et al. Oxygen desaturation index from nocturnal oximetry: a sensitive and specific tool to detect sleep-disordered breathing in surgical patients. Anesth Analg 2012;114(5):993–1000.

51. Scott AS, Baltzan MA, Wolkove N. Examination of pulse oximetry tracings to detect obstructive sleep apnea in patients with advanced chronic obstructive pulmonary disease. Can Respir J 2014;21(3):171–5.

52. Bassetti CLA, Randerath W, Vignatelli L, et al. EAN/ERS/ESO/ESRS statement on the impact of sleep disorders on risk and outcome of stroke. Eur Respir J 2020;55(4):1901104.

53. Andres-Blanco AM, Alvarez D, Crespo A, et al. Assessment of automated analysis of portable oximetry as a screening test for moderate-to-severe sleep apnea in patients with chronic obstructive pulmonary disease. PLoS One 2017;12(11):e0188094.

54. Guilleminault C, Connolly S, Winkle R, et al. Cyclical variation of the heart rate in sleep apnea syndrome. Mechanisms, and usefulness of 24 h

electrocardiography as a screening technique. Lancet 1984;1(8369):126–31.

55. Penzel T, McNames J, Murray A, et al. Systematic comparison of different algorithms for apnoea detection based on electrocardiogram recordings. Med Biol Eng Comput 2002;40(4):402–7.

56. Penzel T. Is heart rate variability the simple solution to diagnose sleep apnoea? Eur Respir J 2003; 22(6):870–1.

57. Heneghan C, de Chazal P, Ryan S, et al. Electrocardiogram recording as a screening tool for sleep disordered breathing. J Clin Sleep Med 2008;4(3): 223–8.

58. Pepin JL, Delavie N, Pin I, et al. Pulse transit time improves detection of sleep respiratory events and microarousals in children. Chest 2005;127(3): 722–30.

59. Bar A, Pillar G, Dvir I, et al. Evaluation of a portable device based on peripheral arterial tone for unattended home sleep studies. Chest 2003;123(3): 695–703.

60. O'Donnell CP, Allan L, Atkinson P, et al. The effect of upper airway obstruction and arousal on peripheral arterial tonometry in obstructive sleep apnea. Am J Respir Crit Care Med 2002;166(7):965–71.

61. Dvir I, Adler Y, Freimark D, et al. Evidence for fractal correlation properties in variations of peripheral arterial tone during REM sleep. Am J Physiol Heart Circ Physiol 2002;283(1):H434–9.

62. Yalamanchali S, Farajian V, Hamilton C, et al. Diagnosis of obstructive sleep apnea by peripheral arterial tonometry: meta-analysis. JAMA Otolaryngol Head Neck Surg 2013;139(12):1343–50.

63. Peppard PE, Young T, Barnet JH, et al. Increased prevalence of sleep-disordered breathing in adults. Am J Epidemiol 2013;177(9):1006–14.

64. Cuspidi C, Tadic M, Sala C, et al. Blood pressure non-dipping and obstructive sleep apnea syndrome: a meta-analysis. J Clin Med 2019;8(9):1367.

65. Genta-Pereira DC, Furlan SF, Omote DQ, et al. Non-dipping blood pressure patterns predict obstructive sleep apnea in patients undergoing ambulatory blood pressure monitoring. Hypertension 2018; 72(4):979–85.

66. Crinion SJ, Ryan S, Kleinerova J, et al. Nondipping nocturnal blood pressure predicts sleep apnea in patients with hypertension. J Clin Sleep Med 2019; 15(07):957–63.

67. Marrone O, Bonsignore MR. Blood-pressure variability in patients with obstructive sleep apnea: current perspectives. Nat Sci Sleep 2018;10:229–42.

68. Davies RJ, Jenkins NE, Stradling JR. Effect of measuring ambulatory blood pressure on sleep and on blood pressure during sleep. BMJ 1994; 308(6932):820–3.

69. Davies RJ, Crosby J, Vardi-Visy K, et al. Non-invasive beat to beat arterial blood pressure during non-REM sleep in obstructive sleep apnoea and snoring. Thorax 1994;49(4):335–9.

70. Lazazzera R, Belhaj Y, Carrault G. A new wearable device for blood pressure estimation using Photoplethysmogram. Sensors (Basel) 2019;19(11):2557.

71. Practice parameters for the use of actigraphy in the clinical assessment of sleep disorders. American Sleep Disorders Association. Sleep 1995;18(4):285–7.

72. Morgenthaler T, Alessi C, Friedman L, et al. Practice parameters for the use of actigraphy in the assessment of sleep and sleep disorders: an update for 2007. Sleep 2007;30(4):519–29.

73. Sadeh A, Hauri PJ, Kripke DF, et al. The role of actigraphy in the evaluation of sleep disorders. Sleep 1995;18(4):288–302.

74. Sadeh A. The role and validity of actigraphy in sleep medicine: an update. Sleep Med Rev 2011;15(4):259–67.

75. Martin JL, Hakim AD. Wrist actigraphy. Chest 2011; 139(6):1514–27.

76. Goldstone A, Baker FC, de Zambotti M. Actigraphy in the digital health revolution: still asleep? Sleep 2018;41(9).

77. Marino M, Li Y, Rueschman MN, et al. Measuring sleep: accuracy, sensitivity, and specificity of wrist actigraphy compared to polysomnography. Sleep 2013;36(11):1747–55.

78. Salmi T, Telakivi T, Partinen M. Evaluation of automatic analysis of SCSB, airflow and oxygen saturation signals in patients with sleep related apneas. Chest 1989;96(2):255–61.

79. Zaffaroni A, de Chazal P, Heneghan C, et al. SleepMinder: an innovative contact-free device for the estimation of the apnoea-hypopnoea index. Annu Int Conf Proc IEEE Eng Med Biol Soc 2009;2009:7091–4.

80. Zaffaroni A, Kent B, O'Hare E, et al. Assessment of sleep-disordered breathing using a non-contact bio-motion sensor. J Sleep Res 2013;22(2):231–6.

81. Pallin M, O'Hare E, Zaffaroni A, et al. Comparison of a novel non-contact biomotion sensor with wrist actigraphy in estimating sleep quality in patients with obstructive sleep apnoea. J Sleep Res 2014;23(4):475–84.

82. Crinion SJ, Tiron R, Lyon G, et al. Ambulatory detection of sleep apnea using a non-contact biomotion sensor. J Sleep Res 2020;29(1):e12889.

83. Ko PR, Kientz JA, Choe EK, et al. Consumer sleep technologies: a review of the landscape. J Clin Sleep Med 2015;11(12):1455–61.

84. Penzel T, Schöbel C, Fietze I. New technology to assess sleep apnea: wearables, smartphones, and accessories. F1000Res 2018;7:413.

85. Behar J, Roebuck A, Domingos JS, et al. A review of current sleep screening applications for smartphones. Physiol Meas 2013;34(7):R29–46.

86. O'Donnell C, Ryan S, McNicholas WT. The impact of telehealth on the organization of the health system and integrated care. Sleep Med Clin 2020;15(3): 431–40.

Objective Measures of Cognitive Performance in Sleep Disorder Research

Kamilla Rún Jóhannsdóttir, PhD[a,b,]*, Dimitri Ferretti, MSc[b],
Birta Sóley Árnadóttir, BSc[a,b], María Kristín Jónsdóttir, PhD[a,b,c]

KEYWORDS

- Sleep disorders • Neurocognitive testing • Cognitive domain • Cognition • Cognitive test battery

KEY POINTS

- Neurocognitive tests can provide an important addition to more traditional noncognitive sleep disorder measures.
- The use of neurocognitive testing in the field needs to be based on standardized practices and theory to conclude on and compare findings.
- We offer an extensive overview of empirical findings organized around neurocognitive tests and different cognitive domains.
- We propose neurocognitive tests and approach for future use of objective measures of cognition in sleep disorder research.

INTRODUCTION

In addition to other more traditional sleep measures, neurocognitive assessment provides an important tool for determining the extent of sleep disruption and the general impact it may have on daily activities, as well as evaluating treatment efficacy. Long-standing sleep disorders are known to have deleterious effects on general health,[1] which in turn influences cognitive functioning[2–4] and may, in the long run, undermine occupational performance and social participation, ultimately leading to diminished quality of life.[5,6] Neurocognitive tests offer objective and reliable assessment of patients' status and progress. To date, however, there is no consensus on how to use neurocognitive assessments in sleep disorder research. The concept of cognitive domain has been used rather inconsistently in the field, with a particular domain being assessed through a single process or even very broadly using a variety of tests. Furthermore, the same test may be used to assess two different domains, making it hard to conclude how cognition is impacted by the various sleep disorders. An effective use of neurocognitive assessment must be based on standardized practices and have a firm theoretic basis.

The purpose of this review was to provide a platform for better standardizing the use of neurocognitive assessment in the field. We aim to do this by reviewing empirical results in sleep disorder research on the basis of the tests used and systematically mapping the different tests onto a corresponding cognitive domain. This approach will help to clarify how different cognitive domains and processes are affected by sleep disorders and also how sensitive a particular test is for detecting impairments owing to sleep disruption. We conclude by suggesting neurocognitive tests for future research, classified by domain and the main cognitive processes involved.

The cognitive domains taken into consideration in the present review are motor skills, perceptual skills, processing speed, vigilance/sustained

[a] Department of Psychology, Reykjavik University, Menntavegur 1, Reykjavik 102, Iceland; [b] Reykjavik University Sleep Institute, School of Technology, Reykjavik University, Menntavegur 1, Reykjavik 102, Iceland; [c] Landspitali University Hospital, Reykjavik, Iceland
* Corresponding author. Reykjavik University, Menntavegur 1, Reykjavik 102, Iceland.
E-mail address: kamilla@ru.is

Sleep Med Clin 16 (2021) 575–593
https://doi.org/10.1016/j.jsmc.2021.08.002
1556-407X/21/© 2021 Elsevier Inc. All rights reserved.

attention, selective attention, episodic memory (verbal/nonverbal), executive function (including working memory), reasoning, decision-making, and emotional processing. We acknowledge that these cognitive domains are not fully independent and that there is not a complete consensus on how to classify cognitive abilities.[7] The sleep disorders considered in this review are obstructive sleep apnea (OSA), sleep-related breathing disorders (SRBD), insomnia and restless leg syndrome (RLS). Only studies completed between 2000 and the present date and based on comparing individuals with specific sleep disorders to a healthy control group are included in the current review.

OBJECTIVE MEASURES OF COGNITIVE DOMAINS IN SLEEP DISORDER RESEARCH
Perceptual Skills

Various perceptual tasks have been used in sleep disorders research, including tasks assessing sensation rather than perception (the function of the perceptual system rather than the processing of the sensory input in the brain). For example, studies have shown that people suffering from OSA have an impaired visual field[8] and a decreased ability to detect high-frequency sounds,[9] both an indication of impaired function of the perceptual system. Tests assessing perceptual skills however, are generally based on the detection of a stimulus and its orientation and location in space.[10] Such tests include the Visual Organization Test and the Judgment of Line Orientation. In a review by Fulda and Schulz,[11] no differences were found in perceptual skills between SRBD and normal controls, evaluated on tests such as Visual Organization Test, Thurstone Visual Matching Test, Judgment of Line Orientation, and the Physical Match and Sensory Motor task. In a recent meta-analysis, perceptual skills were found to be mildly affected by insomnia when assessed with tasks such as the Perceptual Reasoning Index and the Critical Flicker Fusion.[12]

In sum, it is unclear to what extent perceptual skills are affected by sleep disorders. This aspect of neurocognitive functioning is rarely included in studies examining the impact of sleep disorder[13,14] or sleep deprivation[15] on cognitive performance. Yet, impaired perceptual skills, although not perhaps a problem in itself for individuals with sleep disorders, might impact higher order cognitive operations such as attentional control or updating information in working memory (eg, Kilgore[15]). More work is needed in the field to conclude on the impact sleep disorders may have on perceptual skills. Future studies should clearly distinguish between tasks measuring the

function of a perceptual system (sensation) and the perceptual processing of sensory stimuli (perceptual skills).

Motor Skills

Motor skills refer to motor coordination, dexterity and speed.[16] A wide variety of tests have been used to examine motor skills, also referred to as psychomotor function in sleep disorder research (eg, Devita et al[17] and Kilpinen et al[18]). These assessments include tests measuring fine motor coordination and motor speed such as the Mirror Tracing Task, Line Tracing, Rotary Pursuit Test, Finger Tapping Test, the Motor Sequence Learning Task, the Grooved Pegboard, the Purdue Pegboard Test, as well as various simple reaction time tests. Other tests perhaps more suited to assess attention and/or vigilance have also been used as an assessment of motor skills or information processing speed in the field. Note that the Psychomotor Vigilance Test (PVT) measures primarily vigilance and should not be used as an assessment of motor skills.

Ferini-Strambi and colleagues[19] found significantly slower reaction times for individuals with OSA compared with controls on a simple reaction time test. Devita and colleagues[17] used a computerized reaction time test where they distinguished between the perceptual component of reacting to stimuli (the time difference between stimuli appearing and removing a finger from a rest button) and the motor component (the time difference between removing a finger from a rest button and pressing a reaction button). In their study, individuals with OSA had significantly slower reaction times for the motor component in various different reaction time tests compared with normal controls. Khassawneh and colleagues[20] found no significant difference in performance on a simple reaction time test when comparing individuals with insomnia to a control group.

Studies have found impairments in motor speed, coordination, and dexterity for individuals with OSA compared with normal controls using the Purdue Pegboard Test.[19,21] Accordingly, in a review by Fulda and Schulz[11] and Aloia and colleagues,[22] a significantly impaired performance was found on the Purdue Pegboard Test for both individuals with SRBD and individuals with OSA compared with control groups. No impairment, however, was reported for individuals with insomnia on this task.[11,23] Furthermore, no impairment was reported in individuals with various sleep disorders for Finger Tapping Test, Grooved Pegboard, Sensory Motor Task, and Line Tracing Task in 2 reviews.[11,24] Rouleau and colleagues[24] found no difference between individuals with OSA and a normal control group using the Rotary Pursuit Task and the Mirror Tracing Task, although more individuals in the OSA group seemed to have problems during the initial acquisition state of the latter task. Mathieu and colleagues[25] found that age rather than OSA explained differences in performance on the Mirror Tracing Task when comparing younger and older individuals with OSA. However, Neu and colleagues[26] found that individuals with OSA performed significantly worse on Finger Tapping compared with individuals with chronic fatigue syndrome. Similarly, Landry and colleagues[27] found that individuals with OSA demonstrated less learning on Finger Tapping compared with controls after an overnight sleep.

In sum, motor skills as assessed with simple reaction time tests, Finger Tapping, and the Purdue Pegboard, are impaired in individuals with OSA. There is, however, little evidence of impaired motors skills in individuals with insomnia, or in sleep disorders in general for various other motor skills tasks listed elsewhere in this article. More work is needed in the field to gain a comprehensive understanding of the impact sleep disorders may have on motor skills. Impaired motor skills may interfere with performance on tasks measuring executive function or selective attention. Both the Finger Tapping Test and the Purdue Pegboard Test are validated and reliable measures of motor skills.[16] These tests have been suggested as tools for evaluating professionals where coordination, motor speed, and dexterity is important.[28] For example, Ayalon and Friedman[29] found that shift work in resident doctors affected their performance on the Purdue Pegboard Test. Future studies should consider using the Finger Tapping Test, the Purdue Pegboard Test, or some variations of simple reaction time tests when evaluating the impact sleep disorders may have on motor skills.

Processing Speed

Processing speed refers to the ability to rapidly process information and perform various tasks (from simple to complex) such as symbol coding tasks, and connecting numbers/letters in a sequence (Trail Making Tests A), where participants must complete the task as fast as possible.[16] Several studies have shown that individuals with OSA perform worse on the Digit Symbol Substitution Test compared with controls.[24,30–32] A comprehensive review by Kilpinen and colleagues[18] on the impact of OSA on information processing speed measured with tasks such as the Trail Making Test A and the Digit

Symbol Substitution, along with motor control and pursuit tasks, showed a general slowing of information processing speed and psychomotor functions for individuals with OSA compared with control groups. Other studies, however, have found no difference between individuals with OSA and controls for the Trail Making Test A[32] and the Digit Symbol Substitution.[33,34] In the study by Saunamäki and colleagues[33] and Twigg and colleagues,[34] a larger number of individuals in each group was used (n = 40–60) with the age ranging from approximately 20 to 70 years. No difference was found on the Digit Symbol Substitution or the Trail Making Test A when comparing individuals with insomnia (medicated and not) with a control group.[23]

In sum, the studies reviewed in this article are almost entirely focused on OSA and processing speed. In general, there is some indication that processing speed, in particular as measured with the Digit Symbol Substitution, is affected by OSA, but there is insufficient empirical evidence to conclude on other sleep disorders. However, studies have shown that depriving normal individuals of sleep does impair their performance on Digit Symbol Substitution.[35] Furthermore, given the central importance of processing speed for efficient cognitive functioning,[36] it is important to continue studying processing speed in sleep disorders. Also, it should be borne in mind that tests of processing speed are generally confounded by motor speed (eg, the Digit Symbol Substitution Test and the Trail Making Test A) and therefore it is important to use alternative tasks of processing speed that are nonmotor, such as inspection time.[37]

Vigilance and Sustained Attention

Vigilance is the cognitive domain along with executive function that seems to be most affected by sleep disorders.[38–40] Vigilance refers to the ability to sustain attention over time and maintain alertness toward stimuli in the most immediate environment occurring at irregular intervals.[41] Deficits in vigilance caused by sleep deprivation include difficulties sustaining attention over time during continuous task performance, pauses in response time toward stimuli in the task environment (lapses), and response errors (responding too soon, pressing for too long, or missing the target altogether).[42] According to meta-analyses, vigilance is significantly impaired by various sleep disorders such as OSA, indicated by a large effect size.[38] Other reviews and meta-analyses have confirmed that vigilance is significantly affected by OSA (eg, Olaithe and Bucks[39] and Gagnon et al[40]). Decreased vigilance can lead to impairment in other more higher order cognitive functions, such as executive control.[40]

Vigilance is frequently measured with tasks such as the PVT, Continuous Performance Test, Choice Reaction Time Test, and Four Choice Reaction Time Test. Several studies have found impaired performance on the PVT test for individuals with OSA compared with control groups.[43–45] However, Djonlagi and colleagues[46] had different results, with OSA showing no impairment in performance on PVT compared with a control group. Both Li and colleagues[45] and Batool-Anwar and colleagues[43] found that worse performance on the PVT (more lapses and higher reaction times) for individuals with OSA correlated with increased subjective daytime sleepiness as measured with the Epworth Sleepiness Scale. Sforza and colleagues[47] found that errors (lapses and omissions) correlated significantly with both the apnea–hypopnea index and daytime sleepiness in individuals with SRBD. Lee and colleagues[6] found that performance on PVT (lapses and mean reaction times) correlated with quality-of-life measures, in particular, the physical domain for individuals with OSA. This finding was true even after controlling for body mass index, age, apnea severity, and depression. Mathieu and colleagues[25] examining younger and older participants and comparing OSA with a control group, found that individuals with OSA had longer reaction times on Four Choice Reaction Time Test and more lapses compared with controls. For the younger participants with OSA, increased time spent with oxygen saturation of less than 90% caused an increase in reaction time and lapses on the task.

In a large community cohort study,[48] performance on PVT (response speed, not error) varied with the severity of insomnia for older individuals (>65 years). Hansen and colleagues[49] found that PVT differentiated between individuals with sleep-onset insomnia and a control group during a total sleep deprivation period of 39 hours. With an increased number of hours during the sleep deprivation, vigilance as measured with lapses, response errors, and mean reaction time on PVT decreased significantly more for the insomnia group compared with controls. The exaggerated impact of sleep deprivation on individuals with insomnia was found both for the 10-minute version of the PVT and for a 3-minute version. Altena and colleagues[50] used a variation of the PVT, where participants responded to asterisks appearing on a computer screen at random time intervals (the simple vigilance task) and to a target letter (d) ignoring distractors (p) appearing also randomly (complex version). Their results showed that individuals with insomnia did not make more errors, but showed impaired response speed in the complex version compared with a control group, although no difference was found between the two groups in the simple version. Other studies have not found any impairment in performance for individuals with insomnia on Choice Reaction Time Test/Four Choice Reaction Time Test,[20,23] Continuous Performance Test,[51] alertness as measured with the Attention Network Test[52] and on an auditory PVT, both simple and complex.[53]

In sum, there is strong empirical evidence for impaired vigilance and sustained attention in individuals with OSA. It is less clear to what extent vigilance and sustained attention is impaired in individuals with insomnia or other sleep disorders. Interestingly, for insomnia, studies show impaired performance on the original PVT, but not on other measures of vigilance. The PVT has been deemed as perhaps one of the most sensitive measure of the neurocognitive impact of sleep deprivation.[54] The high signal load and the relatively short task performance time makes the PVT test ideal for detecting the impact of insufficient or nonrestorative sleep on vigilance.[54] In addition, research has shown that the short (3-minute) version of the PVT is comparable with the longer 10-minute version in detecting the possible impact of lack of sleep on vigilance.[55,56] The short 3-minute version of the PVT may be ideal for testing elderly and vulnerable patient populations and for repeated testing.

SELECTIVE ATTENTION

Several reviews and meta-analyses have concluded that selective attention is significantly affected by sleep disorders.[22,38,39] However, studies in the field frequently use vigilance measures or executive function measures to examine attention, making it difficult to conclude about selective attention. As pointed out by Strauss and colleagues,[16] it is hard to distinguish attentional selection in space from other cognitive processes such as perception, memory, and motor control. Tests of selective attention include Cancellation tasks, Visual Search tasks, the Posner paradigm, and the Induced Change Blindness task. In all these tests, participants are required to detect an item, object, or area in space, often located among distractors.

Giora and colleagues[13] used a Visual Search task when comparing individuals with OSA to a control group. Participants looked for a target letter (T) appearing among distractors (L, X, O) that varied in number. Their results showed a slower reaction time for individuals with OSA compared with a control group, although search accuracy did not differ between the groups. Similarly, in Giora and colleagues,[14] individuals with insomnia did not differ from a control group in terms of search accuracy on the Visual Search task, but had significantly longer reaction times. Using the Posner paradigm, Woods and colleagues[57] found a significant difference in performance between participants with insomnia and normal sleepers. In their study, the participants with insomnia had a delayed reaction time on invalid trials of the task (ie, the target is not presented at the same side of a computer screen as the cue). Both Jones and colleagues[58] and Marchetti and colleagues[59] using the Induced Change Blindness, found selective attention impairments in patients with insomnia. In the Induced Change Blindness paradigm, a set of flickers is presented to the participant who then has to detect a change, either neutral (a neutral item missing from a picture) or sleep related (eg, a slipper missing from a picture), between the two flickers. In the study done by Marchetti and colleagues,[59] participants with insomnia had a clear bias in their selective attention by being significantly quicker to detect a change related to sleep, but significantly slower to detect a neutral change compared with a control group. Jones and colleagues[58] showed similar results, with individuals with insomnia being quicker to detect a sleep-related change but slower to detect a neutral change compared with normal controls. Although, Rouleau and colleagues[24] found a significant impairment in performance on a cancellation task for individuals with OSA compared with controls, Ferini-Strambi and colleagues[19] found no differences in performance on a cancellation task when comparing OSA to a healthy control group. Khassawneh and colleagues[20] used the Big Circle–Little Circle task to measure selective attention. In this task, participants respond to 1 of 2 circles, responding first to the smaller circle and then to the larger one. No difference was found in performance between individuals with insomnia and a control group.

In sum, very few studies have actually examined selective attention in relation to sleep disorders. In fact, many studies claiming to assess attention are rather assessing attentional control and/or vigilance. Using the Induced Change Blindness task, studies have found attentional bias in individuals with insomnia who respond faster than normal controls to sleep-related changes but slower to neutral changes. There is also some indication that individuals with insomnia have a harder time disengaging attention from a selected area, as demonstrated using the Posner paradigm. Furthermore, individuals with OSA have been found to do worse on a Cancellation task and a Visual Search task. Tasks such as Visual Search are rarely used to assess selective attention, although Wermes and colleagues[60] concluded that reaction times in Visual Search is a reliable measure of selective attention. Future studies should use some of the tasks reviewed in this section when studying the impact that sleep disorders may have on selective attention, avoiding the potential confound with vigilance and executive control. The benefit of the Induce Blindness paradigm is that the task does not confound target detection with motor control.

Executive Function and Working Memory

Executive function refers to various top-down processes that regulate and control cognitive performance by guiding attention, updating information in working memory, overseeing attentional switching between tasks and inhibiting untimely or inappropriate responses.[61–63] It is currently widely accepted that executive functions include three main domains: (1) maintenance of information in working memory and updating of that information, (2) inhibitory control (including the control of attention), and (3) cognitive flexibility or set shifting.[61,63] For the most part, recent research on cognition in sleep disorders divides executive function into the three recognized domains (see Ballesio et al[64]). However, in the literature as a whole, a variety of tasks are used to evaluate executive function, many of which are more suitable for evaluating other domains, such as attention, processing speed, or vigilance. Both reviews and meta-analyses indicate strongly that executive function is impaired by various sleep disorders, such as OSA,[40,65] linking OSA with impairment in working memory, inhibitory control, and cognitive flexibility.[65] In a meta-analysis by Fortier-Brochue and associates,[66] insomnia had a significant impact on the working memory part of executive function (eg, maintaining, updating and manipulating information) while inhibitory control and cognitive flexibility were less affected.

Working memory

Recognized working memory tasks that have been used in sleep disorder research include, the Backward Digit Span,[67] the Corsi Block Test, and the N-back Test.[68] Both the Backward Digit Span and the Corsi Block Test are among the most frequently used tests when evaluating the impact sleep disorders may have on working memory.[65] Other tests used include Double Span Memory Task, and the Paced Auditory Serial Addition Test.[69]

Torelli and colleagues[70] found that individuals with OSA performed significantly worse on the Backward Digit Span than controls. Other studies, however, do not show an impaired performance on the Backward Digit Span when comparing individuals with OSA with a control group.[19,25,32,33,71] In the study by Torelli and colleagues,[70] only 16 individuals with OSA participated and most of them (n = 12) had severe OSA. Ferini-Strambi and colleagues[19] found no difference in performance on the Corsi Block Test and Canessa and colleagues[72] found no difference on the N-back Test when comparing individuals with OSA with control groups. Thomas and colleagues,[73] however, testing young individuals with OSA compared with controls, found that individuals with OSA had slower performance speed and less accuracy in the N-back Test. Using a comprehensive selection of working memory tests, Naëgelé and colleagues[74] found that individuals with OSA were not impaired on short-term span measures or dual task measures. They did, however, find a significantly impaired performance for individuals with OSA on the Paced Auditory Serial Addition Test, which is a highly speeded task, and on a modified Auditory Span task, where participants have to maintain a list of numbers as well as perform simple arithmetic transformation on the numbers.

In contrast with studies on OSA, studies on individuals with insomnia show a marked impairment in working memory. Both Haimov and colleagues[75] and Vignola and colleagues[23] found that performance on the Backward Digit Span was significantly impaired for individuals with insomnia. Similarly, Cellini and colleagues[76] found that young individuals with insomnia had a higher number of errors and less total accuracy on N-back compared with controls. Shekleton and colleagues[53] also found impaired performance on the N-back Test among individuals with insomnia and short sleep duration; no difference in performance on the task was found for insomnia with normal sleep duration compared with controls. Lovato and colleagues[77] found no significant difference between older individuals with insomnia and controls on the Double Span Memory task when controlling for IQ.

Inhibitory control

Accepted neurocognitive tasks for measuring inhibitory control that are also used frequently in the field of sleep disorder research include the Stroop Test (also the Color–Word Interference Test), the Simon task,[78] the Flanker Test,[79] the Go/No Go,[80] and the Stop Signal task.[81] These tasks not only require the individual to inhibit unwanted responses, but also to direct attention to the relevant task-related goal. When performing on the tasks the participant needs to respond to particular information (direction or color of stimuli) while ignoring other information (location or reading words). In the Go/No Go and the Stop Signal tasks, the focus is more on the inhibition of response.[63] The participant must respond to stimuli (eg, letters) as fast as possible but refrain from responding to a particular stimulus or when a cue is given at random intervals. Outcome measures include accuracy and reaction time as well as stop signal reaction time.

Individuals with OSA have been shown to have impaired performance on the Stroop Test (increased error, not time) and the Flanker Test.[19,71,82] In a Canadian longitudinal study on aging with a large cohort, individuals with insomnia disorders (>45 years of age, n = 1068) did worse on the Stroop Test than those with no insomnia (n = 19,604) and insomnia symptoms only (n = 7813) after controlling for age, education, and sex.[83] Similarly, other studies have found a significantly impaired performance for individuals with insomnia (compared with control groups) on the Stroop Test[75] and the Flanker Test.[52] Other studies have not found a significant difference in performance on the Stroop Test for insomnia[84] or RLS.[85]

Covassin and colleagues[86] compared eight individuals with insomnia with eight good sleepers, using the Stop Signal task. They found that the individuals with insomnia had a harder time inhibiting their responses when the auditory cue was given. Studies have similarly found that both individuals with OSA[87] and insomnia[88] have a harder time preventing their responses to the no go stimuli. In contrast, Sagaspe and colleagues[87] found no difference in performance for individuals with insomnia and Angelelli and colleagues[89] found no difference in performance for individuals with OSA compared with a control group on the Go/No Go task. Mean age of participants was similar between the studies, but both Zhao and colleagues[88] and Covassin and colleagues[86] had very few participants (n < 15).

Cognitive flexibility (switching)

Recognized tests used to measure cognitive flexibility and also used in sleep disorder research include the Wisconsin Card Sorting Test, Trail Making Test B, and various attentional switching tasks such as the Task Switching Paradigm and the Switching to Attention Test. Werli and colleagues[71] found a significant difference between individuals with OSA and controls on both categories and perseverative errors on the Wisconsin

Card Sorting Test (see also Rouleau et al[24]). Other studies have, however, not found a difference on the Wisconsin Card Sorting Test when comparing individuals with OSA with healthy control groups.[25,90] de Almondes and colleagues[91] found no difference between individuals with insomnia and controls on the test (see also Vignola et al[23]). Similarly, no differences were found by Fang and colleagues[92] on the Wisconsin Card Sorting Test when comparing individuals with insomnia and control participants despite objective measures showing a difference in total sleep time and less sleep efficiency for individuals with insomnia. Although Ju and colleagues[93] found that individuals with OSA were significantly slower to complete the Trail Making Test B compared with a healthy control group and made more errors, other studies have not found any performance impairments on Trail Making Test B for individuals with OSA.[19,25,32,71,94] Similarly, no performance impairment on Trail Making Test B has been found for insomnia[23,84] or individuals with RLS.[85,95]

In the switching tasks such as the Task Switching Paradigm and Switching to Attention Test, both attentional switching and response inhibition are evaluated.[96] Participants are required to switch between different tasks, for example, judging if a number is odd or even, and bigger or smaller than the number 5 in Task Switching Paradigm (eg, Sdoia and Ferlazzo[96] and Wilckens et al[97]) and switch between location and direction of arrows in Switching to Attention Test.[51] Which task the participant has to work on is indicated by a cue such as the shape of geometric figures (eg, Ballesio and colleagues[64] and Wilckens and colleagues[97]). Performing according to the same task rule results in a faster reaction times compared with when the participant switches from one task to another, this is referred to as switching cost.[96] In a study by Wilckens and colleagues,[97] older patients with insomnia were significantly worse in using a preparation time (time between cue and target) compared with a control group. Similarly, Shekleton and colleagues[53] found that patients with insomnia were significantly slower compared with controls to respond to the stimuli in the complex switching condition of the Switching to Attention Test (switching between location and direction). Interestingly, Shekleton and colleagues[53] found that only individuals with insomnia who reported short total sleep time (<6 hours) showed worse performance on the Switching to Attention Test compared with a control group but not those who reported longer total sleep time (>6 hours). Khassawneh and colleagues[20] found that individuals with insomnia and objectively measured short total sleep time (<6 hours) showed significantly higher response latency and errors on the Switching to Attention Test compared with a normal control group. However, Ballesio and colleagues[98] did not find impaired performance on Task Switching Paradigm after partial sleep deprivation (5 hours of sleep) for patients with chronic insomnia compared with controls.

Verbal Fluency tests and the Maze test are also frequently used to assess cognitive flexibility.[63] In the fluency tests, participants are asked to produce as many words starting with a particular letter (phonemic fluency) or members of a particular category (semantic fluency) as they can for a given time period.[16,63,99] Both Ferini-Strambi and colleagues[19] and Salorio and colleagues[90] found a significantly impaired performance in individuals with OSA compared with controls for phonemic, but not semantic fluency. Werli and colleagues,[71] however, found that individuals with OSA did significantly worse on both semantic and phonemic fluency tests compared with controls. Other studies have not found any differences in phonemic fluency[24,70,74] or semantic fluency[70,93] for OSA compared with controls. Sivertsen and colleagues[84] found a significantly impaired performance for older individuals with insomnia on phonemic but not semantic fluency test. Pearson and colleagues[85] compared 16 individuals diagnosed with RLS with a matched control group and found that individuals with RLS had a significantly impaired performance on a semantic fluency test compared with controls. Other studies have not found any differences for Verbal Fluency for RLS.[95] Impaired performance on the Maze Test has been reported for individuals with OSA,[24] but not for individuals with RLS.[85]

In sum, various reviews and meta-analyses indicate a strong impact of sleep disorders on executive function.[38,65] In fact, it has been concluded that executive functioning is the aspect of cognition that is most heavily impacted by sleep disorders.[39] Accordingly, it is clear from the present review that there are some impairments in executive function among individuals with sleep disorders. However, measures need to be chosen carefully and in order to conclude whether or not a particular sleep disorder affects executive function, all three domains must be examined (working memory, inhibition and control, and cognitive flexibility). When it comes to impaired working memory, the results were more conflicted for OSA than for insomnia. Individuals with insomnia show impaired performance on all working memory tasks. However, most studies on working memory and OSA show no performance impairment in particular those studies using the

Backward Digit Span. In a comprehensive study by Naëgelé and colleagues,[74] OSA seemed to have little impact on short-term span or dual task working memory measures, but greater impact on more fast paced complex working memory tasks such as the Paced Auditory Serial Addition Test and the Auditory Span task.

Inhibition and attentional control are impaired in individuals with OSA and individuals with insomnia. Tests such as the Stroop Test and the Flanker Test may be a good option for detecting this impairment in sleep disorders. For cognitive flexibility, studies using both the Wisconsin Card Sorting Test and the Trail Making Test B show no clear differences in performance of individuals with OSA, individuals with insomnia, and individuals with RLS compared with control groups. Both the Wisconsin Card Sorting Test and the Trail Making Test B are very popular and frequently used tests in clinical assessment but they may be more sensitive to serious frontal lobe problems rather then to the performance decrement caused by sleep disorders.[64] When measuring cognitive flexibility, switching tasks may be a better option in sleep disorder research. Studies have shown that individuals with insomnia have a harder time switching between tasks compared with normal controls. The results for fluency tasks are very conflicted for OSA, insomnia, and RLS. Although studies vary in terms of the number of participants and age, no systematic differences were found in demographics between studies that could explain the difference in results.

Episodic Memory (Verbal and Nonverbal)

Episodic memory refers to memory for particular events, recent as well as in the more distant past that are tied to time and place.[100] It is normally tested by measuring both immediate and delayed verbal and visual recall using both recognition and free recall.[11,40] Measures also include learning when participants, for example, go repeatedly through the same word list. A variety of verbal memory tests exists and have been used in the field of sleep disorder research. The Auditory Verbal Learning Test tests immediate and delayed recall of semantically unrelated words.[16] In Logical Memory (the Wechsler Memory Scale), participants need to store and retrieve information from a story and in both the California Verbal Learning Test and the Hopkins Verbal Learning Test, participants work with semantically related information.[101] There is also the Verbal Paired Associates Test.[101] Meta-analyses and reviews indicate impaired verbal memory in OSA[102] and insomnia.[12] In fact, Wallace and Bucks[102]

concluded that all aspects of verbal memory are impaired in individuals with OSA, that is, immediate and delayed recall as well as recognition and learning. According to Fulda and Schultz,[11] there is little indication of memory impairment in insomnia and SRBD.

Naëgelé and colleagues[74] used 16-word word lists where participants had to identify the category of each word as they went through the list (individuals with OSA compared with controls). They then tested immediate recall before and after an interfering task and a cued recall (repeated 3 times). The participants also completed a recognition test and a delayed free recall test. In general, individuals with OSA performed on par with normal controls, except on immediate free recall after interference. The authors concluded that impaired memory in individuals with OSA is isolated to the retrieval process, not the encoding, learning, or retention parts of verbal memory. Using a word list and immediate and delayed recall, Ju and colleagues[93] also found that immediate and delayed free recall is impaired for older individuals with OSA compared with controls, but not recognition memory. Other studies using the Auditory Verbal Learning Test have also found that individuals with OSA perform worse than controls.[26,70,71,103,104] Werli and colleagues[71] found only a difference in the delayed free recall of the Auditory Verbal Learning Test, whereas Neu and colleagues[26] found a difference in both immediate and delayed free recall when comparing OSA with controls. Neither study found any difference in recognition. Other studies have, however, not found any performance difference on the Auditory Verbal Learning Test when comparing individuals with OSA with controls.[24,25,84,105] Using the California Verbal Learning Test, Salorio and colleagues[90] found a significantly impaired overall recall, but not in retention for OSA compared with a control group.

Adams and colleagues[106] found that SRBD correlated with performance on the California Verbal Learning Test. Similarly, Cross and colleagues[83] found a significantly worse performance on the Auditory Verbal Learning Test, both immediate and delayed recall, in a large population-based cohort comparing insomniacs with controls. However, Sivertsen and colleagues[84] found no difference in performance on California Verbal Learning Test for older insomniacs compared with controls. In a study by Guo and colleagues[3] comparing insomniacs with controls, participants read out loud a list of object-related words and were then tested immediately and after a 5 minute delay (free recall) and again after a 20-minute delay (recognition). The results showed that individuals with insomnia were significantly worse at immediate and delayed free recall, but no difference was between the groups on the delayed recognition test. Vignola and colleagues[23] found no differences in individuals with insomnia compared with controls on immediate and delayed memory on the verbal paired associates test.

Using the Logical Memory Test, Mathieu and colleagues[25] found a significant difference in both immediate and delayed recall for individuals with OSA compared with control for both younger and older individuals. Similarly, Twigg and colleagues[34] found that individuals with OSA had impaired immediate and delayed recall compared with normal controls, but their recognition memory and maintaining information over time was intact. Ferini-Strambi and colleagues,[19] however, with fewer participants (n = 23 vs 60) found no difference between individuals with OSA and controls on the Logical Memory Test.

Studies suggest that immediate and delayed recall in visual memory is impaired in individuals with OSA.[102] Tests used to assess nonverbal memory include the Rey-Osterrieth Complex Figure, the Brief Visuospatial Memory Test,[101] the Wechsler Memory Scale (Visual Reproduction, Figural Memory, Visuospatial Delayed Recall and Visual Memory Test),[107] and the Wechsler Adult Intelligence Scale-Revised (Block Design). In the Visual Memory Test, participants are asked to recognize a target picture among distractors after viewing it briefly. Torelli and colleagues[70] found no significant difference in individuals with OSA compared with controls on the Visual Memory Test. In the Rey-Osterrieth Complex Figure Test, participants are asked to copy a complex figure and then reproduce the same figure from memory twice (immediate and delayed memory). Some studies have found that both individuals with SRBD[104,106] and those with OSA[24,70] perform worse on the Rey-Osterrieth Complex Figure Test compared with normal controls. However, other studies have not found any significant differences in performance.[19,34,84] Daurat and colleagues[108] found that the recollection of temporal and spatial memories is impaired in patients with OSA using the Brief Visuospatial Memory Test Revised. In the Wechsler Memory Scale Visual Reproduction subtest,[107] participants are shown visual designs and later asked to draw the designs as they remember them (immediate and delayed recall). Vignola and colleagues[23] found no difference in performance here for individuals with insomnia compared with controls.

In sum, it is clear that for verbal memory there is an impairment in both immediate and delayed free recall for individuals with OSA but not in retention of information, because their performance on recognition tests seems intact. Similarly, although less empirical evidence exists on verbal memory in insomnia, individuals with insomnia also seem to do worse on recall than on recognition tests. The evidence for impairment in nonverbal (visual) memory is less clear than the evidence for verbal memory problems and warrants further investigation. Studies reviewed here tend not to show any impairments in performance on nonverbal tests for individuals with sleep disorders; however, it is possible that the difference between impairments in verbal and nonverbal recall is the greater emphasis on attentional processes in verbal tasks, such as list recall.

Reasoning, Decision-Making, and Emotional Processing

Reasoning refers to logical thinking and judgment[101] and can be measured with tests such as the Wechsler Adult Intelligence Scale (eg, Matrix Reasoning and Picture Arrangement subtests), the Ravens Progressive Matrices, and Colored Progressive Matrices. Reasoning is rarely included in reviews and meta-analysis in the field because it is seldom included in studies on cognition in sleep disorders. According to Fulda and Schulz,[11] no conclusion can be drawn regarding reasoning in SRBD owing to scarce evidence. In the Raven's test, participants need to choose visual design items from a set of distractors that logically fit in a given visual set. Studies have reported no impairment in performance on the Raven's test for individuals with OSA compared with controls.[19,70] In a study by Sivertsen and colleagues,[84] no differences were found in performance on Matrix Reasoning when comparing individuals with insomnia with controls. Furthermore, Pearson and colleagues[85] found no differences in performance on the Colored Progressive Matrices when comparing RLS with controls.

Although generally not included in meta-analyses and reviews, decision-making in relation to sleep disorders has been studied quite extensively and sleep deprivation in normal individuals has been found to impair decision-making under uncertainty.[109,110] The tasks used to assess decision-making, include, the Iowa Gambling Test, Game of Dice Task, Balloon Analog Risk Task, and the Bead Task.

In the Iowa Gambling Test, the individual's ability to learn from the consequences of the card selected and adapt his or her decision-making strategies accordingly is evaluated.[111] Cards are presented on a computer screen; one-half of them are advantageous (smaller rewards and smaller losses) and one-half are disadvantageous (large rewards but also occasional large losses). Most participants learn that, in the long run, choosing the advantageous cards is beneficial. Examining untreated individuals with OSA, Delazer and colleagues[94] found no difference between individuals with OSA and a healthy control group when looking at the performance on the Iowa Gambling Test. The individuals with OSA showed an average performance, where they learned from the consequences of their card selection and over time selected more the advantageous cards over the disadvantageous cards, as did the healthy control group. Interestingly, however, when looking at the performance of the individuals, more individuals in the OSA group (13%) showed impaired performance (choosing the risky cards) compared with the healthy control group. Daurat and colleagues[112] found that individuals with OSA tended to select the risky decks significantly more frequently than a normal control group. McNally and colleagues[113] found a decreased learning effect during the Iowa Gambling Test for individuals with a higher risk of SRBD compared with lower risk individuals and healthy controls. In Chunhua and colleagues,[114] individuals with insomnia showed less sensitivity to the risky cards in the Iowa Gambling Test compared with a control group. Their results showed that, for the first round of card playing, there was no difference between those with insomnia and the control group. However, after the first round of card playing the individuals with insomnia selected significantly fewer cards from the advantageous card deck compared with healthy controls, suggesting that they had a harder time learning from the consequences of their card selection.

To evaluate decision-making abilities in subjects with RLS, Bayard and colleagues[115,116] used both the Iowa Gambling Test and the Game of Dice Task. In the Game of Dice Task, the participants are asked to maximize their income through a series of dice throws choosing between single numbers or combination for each throw. Both studies[115,116] showed worse performances for individuals with RLS for the Iowa Gambling Test (showing a more risk-oriented decisions), but not for the Game of Dice Task (where probabilities are calculable).

On the Balloon Analog Risk Task, participants are requested to inflate a digital balloon or collect a reward. After each inflate the amount the participant gains in a reward increases and can be lost if the balloon explodes.[117] Higher scores show a greater risk-taking propensity.[118] There is some indication that poor sleep quality may cause individuals to become less risk oriented on the Balloon Analog Risk Task.[119] However, other studies have not found any impact of partial sleep loss on performance on the task.[120] Several studies using the Bead Task have shown impaired decision-making in patients with RLS (eg, Heim et al[121,122]). In the Beads Task, participants are shown two cups of colored beads, one with mainly blue beads and another with mainly green beads. They are then asked to estimate from which cup a bead is drawn (the participant can wait a certain number of draws before giving an answer, the best strategy is to wait as much as possible instead of just "jump to the conclusion"). Participants are also informed about the cost in dollars for an incorrect choice of urn. The percentage of colors can vary between tasks (eg, 60/40 or 80/20) and before any draw the participant is informed about the distribution in percentage of beads in the two urns.[123,124] In the study from Heim and colleagues,[121] individuals with RLS tended to jump to conclusion more than the control group. Similar results can be found in a another study,[122] where individuals with RLS showed a more impulsive behavior on the bead task than a control group, asking for fewer trials and giving answers with less information. Similar results were found in a recent study,[125] where more impulsive behavior was found in individuals with RLS (with augmentation and augmentation plus impulse control disorder) compared to healthy controls.

McNally and colleagues[113] suggest that the Iowa Gambling Test could be a sensitive task (in sleep pathology) owing to the double valence of the task, both in decision-making and also in emotional functioning. In fact, studies have found impaired emotional processing with sleep-deprived individuals rating neutral stimuli more negatively compared with rested individuals[126,127] and also demonstrating increased emotional sensitivity and decreased emotional empathy.[114,128] Heinrich and colleagues[119] found that induced hypoxia and poor sleep cause impaired emotions recognition. Almost no work has been done on examining emotional processing in sleep disorders. However, in one study[46] individuals with OSA rated their self-perceived mood more negatively than controls. Chunhua and colleagues[114] found no difference between individuals with insomnia and control in evaluating emotional pictures; however, on a delayed recognition task the individuals with insomnia did worse in general but tended to remember better negative than positive and neutral pictures. de Almodes and colleagues[91] found that individuals with insomnia had impaired recognition of facial expression of sadness and fear compared with healthy controls. Furthermore, the impoverished emotional judgment was associated with poor performance on cognitive tests measuring inhibitory control and cognitive flexibility.

In sum, there is no indication of impaired reasoning abilities in sleep disorders, but more work is needed owing to insufficient empirical testing. However, decision-making is impaired in individuals with OSA, insomnia, and RLS. Studies show that individuals with various sleep disorders tend to make more risky choices and do not learn from negative consequences. Accordingly, there is also an indication that emotional processing may be impaired in these individuals, with studies showing that sleep disruption can lead to a bias toward negative emotional stimuli and impaired emotional judgment.

SUMMARY AND FUTURE DIRECTIONS

As summarized elsewhere in this article, numerous studies have established that various sleep disorders can entail cognitive difficulties that present as objectively measurable problems (eg, Wardle-Pinkston et al[12] and Bucks et al[129]), but also as subjective complaints.[12,130] Using neurocognitive measures as objective daytime assessment of sleep disorders can therefore be an important tool in addition to traditional sleep measures. Cognitive measures can be useful to monitor patient progress or decline[131] and predict compliance,[132] as well as providing patients with information about their cognitive status and validating their cognitive complaints.

All the sleep disorders considered in the current review—namely, OSA, SRBD, insomnia, and RLS—have been found to result in cognitive problems at various levels of the cognitive system. According to meta-analyses the cognitive factors most often affected are attention (vigilance), executive functions and memory (eg, Bucks et al[129]). Cognitive components that are not commonly reported are language and visuo-constructional abilities. However, it should be kept in mind that it is hard to reach firm conclusions given the lack of standard practices in neurocognitive testing in the field. As pointed out by Aloia and colleagues,[132] study results are determined by which areas of cognition are assessed and which are left out. Some areas, for example, visuoconstructional abilities, nonverbal memory, and basic perceptual functions, are relatively seldom explored and thus knowledge on how these areas are affected by sleep disorders is incomplete. Thus, domains that are reported to be affected, depend on the choice of tests in each particular study.

More than 20 years ago, Décary and colleagues[133] proposed a neuropsychological test battery to be used in OSA research. However, no particular combination of cognitive test is currently favored in sleep disorder research. Rather, a variety of tests have been used, both standardized clinical tests (eg, the Trail Making Test), as well as tests that have traditionally mostly been used in more basic cognitive research (eg, the Brown–Peterson paradigm). Further, there has not been a systematic review of how to map cognitive tests onto domains of cognition and the concept of cognitive domain has been used rather inconsistently, which certainly is not unique to the sleep disorder field. The concept of cognitive domain has thus been used for a single component of a larger domain such as in Leng and colleagues,[4] where delayed memory is used as a measure of the memory domain and in Wardle-Pinkston and associates,[12] where there are 2 separate working memory components (retention and manipulation). In other studies, the cognitive domains are broader and even include components or tests that elsewhere are allotted to 2 different domains.

The lack of a standard cognitive battery for use in sleep research was discussed by Bucks and colleagues,[129] who made several recommendations. They pointed out, for example, the importance of taking into account the expertise required to administer and interpret cognitive tests and the population of interest (eg, sex, age). However, they did not make specific recommendations regarding particular tests and how various domains should preferably be assessed.

How, then, might the ideal cognitive battery for sleep disorders look? First, one could consider separate batteries for clinical and research use. Research usually requires tests that take less time and that can potentially be administered online, even self-administrated.[134] Further, tests that have alternate versions for repeat testing could also be advantageous. However, this notion also applies to clinical testing. Research tests should also, to the extent possible, stress a single cognitive domain, because there will not be room for clinical interpretation of affected domains and perhaps not the required clinical expertise.[129] In a clinical context, the emphasis may be different as clinical interpretation comes into play.

Another important dimension to consider when choosing tests is age. Similar test batteries may not be appropriate for all ages. In some sleep studies the Mini-Mental State Examination or the Modified Mini-Mental State have been used as a measure of global cognitive function.[4] These tests lack sensitivity in young and otherwise healthy populations, but may be relevant in older populations where general cognitive decline or impending dementia are suspected. The impact general physical

Table 1
Suggested tests for sleep research and their corresponding cognitive domains based on theoretic groupings

Domain	Test[a]	Cognitive Processes[b]
Motor skills	Simple reaction time[139]	Motor speed/reaction time
	Purdue Pegboard Test[101]	Manual dexterity and coordination/speed
Perceptual skills	Line orientation[101]	Visuoperceptual ability, visual matching. spatial relations
	The Benton Visual Form Discrimination test[101]	Visual discrimination
Processing speed	Symbol Search[140]	Processing speed/psychomotor speed/ visual scanning
	Digit Symbol Coding[140]	Processing speed and many others (eg, short-term visual memory, implicit learning, psychomotor speed, visual scanning)
	Inspection time[37]	Nonmotor cognitive speed, perceptual speed, selective attention
Vigilance/sustained attention	PVT[138]	Sustained attention, reaction time
	Choice reaction time[139]	Vigilance/motor speed/reaction time/ decision-making
Selective attention	Cancellation task (eg, Bell test)[101]	Selective attention, scanning, motor speed
	Induced Change Blindness[59]	Selective attention, reaction times
Executive functioning	Corsi blocks[101]/Paced Auditory Serial Addition Test [101]	Maintenance and processing of information in working memory
	Stroop test[101]	Inhibition/attentional control
	Task switching paradigm[97]	Flexibility/set shifting
Visuoconstruction	Copy of Rey-Osterrieth Complex Figure[101]	Visuoconstructive abilities, planning/ executive function, motor speed
Episodic memory	Word list learning (eg, Rey Auditory Verbal Learning)[101]	Verbal memory (learning, immediate and delayed retrieval)
	Rey-Osterrieth Complex Figure - recall[101]	Nonverbal memory (learning, immediate and delayed retrieval)
Language	Naming tests (eg, Boston naming)[101]	Semantic retrieval
	Category Verbal Fluency[101]	Lexical access speed/cognitive speed
	Semantic priming[141]	Semantic memory integrity/motor speed
Reasoning/decision-making	Matrix reasoning (eg, from WAIS-IV).[140]	Visual/perceptual reasoning/attention and concentration
	Iowa Gambling task[113]	Evaluating choices based on consequences/ evaluating risks/decision-making under uncertainty
Global cognition	Addenbrooke test,[142] Montreal Cognitive Assessment[143] (older populations) Wechsler Abbreviated Scale of Intelligence[144] (for younger populations)	Nonspecific – taps into various cognitive factors

[a] Note that in some cases there are several comparable tests available.
[b] These are not complete, but major components are indicated.

health or disease burden can have on cognitive functioning[135] is also particularly relevant in older patients, in which case disentangling the cognitive impact of sleep disorders and other health issues might prove difficult when disease burden is not controlled for. Also, a long-standing sleep disorder is a risk factor for dementia,[136] which further complicates the picture in the elderly.

We propose that, when testing possible cognitive impairments among patients with sleep disorders, it is important to cover cognitive factors at all levels of the cognitive system. Because sleep disorders are likely to have diffuse cognitive effects most, if not all, cognitive domains should be addressed to some degree and more than one test should be used for each domain, because most tests are not pure measures of a single cognitive factor. We fully acknowledge that the various cognitive domains are not fully independent and that there is not a complete consensus on how to classify cognitive abilities into domains.[7] Also, groupings of tests into cognitive domains may depend on whether the groupings are done theoretically or by using factor analysis on a large battery of tests. Furthermore the factor structure may also depend on the populations studied (ie, healthy vs patient populations) (eg, Siedlecki et al[137]). It is important to be cognizant of this issue and be able to address it, for example, in justifying choice of tests and in conceptualizing and interpreting results.

Based on our review and having taken the various levels of cognition and cognitive domains into consideration, tests that are appropriate for sleep disorder research have been listed in **Table 1** along with the domain they belong to.

The list in **Table 1** is not the ultimate and final list of tests to be used in sleep research. Rather, it is presented as a framework and a way to think about cognitive testing in sleep research. Thus, as shown, we present two very different motor tests that assess basic stimulus-reaction times and dexterity that is also speed related. In addition, the cognitive hierarchy is the basis for choosing the test, although it should not be forgotten that the domains intersect. Given the usual time constraints in research, it is unlikely that it is possible to administer all tests in every study. However, we believe that with 90 minutes of testing, sampling from all domains can be done. Given the amount of useful information that can be obtained with cognitive testing this is time well spent.

Many of the tests listed in **Table 1** exist as a part of well-developed psychological tests, such as the Wechsler Intelligence Scales (eg, Digit Symbol Substitution Test and Matrix Reasoning).[145] Others are well-recognized neuropsychological test that have been used for decades in the clinic as well as in research (eg, the Auditory Verbal Learning Test, Rey-Osterrieth Complex Figure, and Purdue Pegboard Test).[101] Others are nonclinical tests (eg, reaction times, semantic priming, and Induced Change Blindness) or both nonclinical and experimental, such as the Iowa Gambling Test. All the tests listed have an extensive literature behind them and are known to be valid and sensitive and the clinical tests have extensive normative literature.[101] Also, many of the tests that are generally used as paper-and-pencil tests have been digitized or can be digitized and run on computers. Further, some of the tests are appropriate for repeat testing and have minimal practice effects (eg, the PVT),[39] although practice effects when testing cognition should always be kept in mind, because they have even been found with simple reaction time tests.[146]

Neurocognitive testing is a complex procedure and goes beyond pure testing. When planning a cognitive test battery, it is important to be aware of the many cognitive processes required for solving what, on the face of it, seems to be a simple cognitive task. This practice will result in a more balanced test battery, which in turn should ease the interpretation of results. In the best of worlds, a standardized neurocognitive battery, used across a variety of sleep disorders and in multiple centers across the world would be ideal. This approach would facilitate comparisons of studies, across disorders and different populations. A standardized battery has been suggested before,[133] but it did not reach the sleep research community as a whole. Perhaps the time is now ripe and we call for a consensus on the use of cognitive measures in sleep research.

CLINICS CARE POINTS

- When using cognitive tests in the clinic, using appropriate normative data, stratified by age and education, is critical.

- Keep in mind that tests such as the Mini-Mental Examination Test, Addenbrooke, and Montreal Cognitive Assessment are only screening tests.

- In the clinic, it is important to distinguish between testing (ie, cognitive screening) and detailed professional neuropsychological evaluation.

- A diagnosis of dementia cannot be based on cognitive assessment only and medical history and other relevant information needs to be integrated with psychological assessment.

DISCLOSURE

The authors have nothing to disclose. The work of the authors is sponsored in part by the Sleep Revolution, which has received funding from the European Union's Horizon 2020 research and innovation programme under grant agreement no. 965417 and by NordForsk (NordSleep project 90458-06111) via the Icelandic Centre for Research.

REFERENCES

1. Shahar E, Whitney CW, Redline S, et al. Sleep-disordered breathing and cardiovascular disease: cross-sectional results of the Sleep Heart Health Study. Am J Respir Crit Care Med 2001;163(1): 19–25.

2. Caporale M, Palmeri R, Corallo F, et al. Cognitive impairment in obstructive sleep apnea syndrome: a descriptive review. Sleep Breath 2021;25(1): 29–40.

3. Guo H, Wei M, Ding W. Changes in cognitive function in patients with primary insomnia. Shanghai Arch Psychiatry 2017;29(3):137–45.

4. Leng Y, McEvoy CT, Allen IE, et al. Association of sleep-disordered breathing with cognitive function and risk of cognitive impairment: a systematic review and meta-analysis. JAMA Neurol 2017; 74(10):1237–45.

5. Brown WD. The psychosocial aspects of obstructive sleep apnea. Semin Respir Crit Care Med 2005;26(1):33–43.

6. Lee I-S, Bardwell W, Ancoli-Israel S, et al. The Relationship between psychomotor vigilance performance and quality of life in obstructive sleep apnea. J Clin Sleep Med 2011;7(3):254–60.

7. Sachdev PS, Blacker D, Blazer DG, et al. Classifying neurocognitive disorders: the DSM-5 approach. Nat Rev Neurol 2014;10(11):634–42.

8. Tsang CSL, Chong SL, Ho CK, et al. Moderate to severe obstructive sleep apnoea patients is associated with a higher incidence of visual field defect. Eye (Lond) 2006;20(1):38–42.

9. Vorlová T, Dlouhá O, Kemlink D, et al. Decreased perception of high frequency sound in severe obstructive sleep apnea. Physiol Res 2016;65(6): 959–67.

10. Farah MJ. Disorders of visual-spatial perception and cognition, . Clinical neuropsychology. 4th Ed. Oxford University Press; 2003. p. 146–60.

11. Fulda S, Schulz H. Cognitive dysfunction in sleep disorders. Sleep Med Rev 2001;5(6):423–45.

12. Wardle-Pinkston S, Slavish DC, Taylor DJ. Insomnia and cognitive performance: a systematic review and meta-analysis. Sleep Med Rev 2019;48: 101205.

13. Giora E, Galbiati A, Marelli S, et al. Evidence of perceptive impairment in OSA patients investigated by means of a visual search task. Cortex 2017;95:136–42.

14. Giora E, Galbiati A, Marelli S, et al. Impaired visual processing in patients with insomnia disorder revealed by a dissociation in visual search. J Sleep Res 2017;26(3):338–44.

15. Killgore WDS. Effects of sleep deprivation on cognition. Prog Brain Res 2010;185:105–29.

16. Strauss E, Sherman EMS, Spreen O. A compendium of neuropsychological tests: administration, norms, and commentary. 3rd edition. New York: Oxford University Press; 2006. p. xvii, 1216.

17. Devita M, Montemurro S, Zangrossi A, et al. Cognitive and motor reaction times in obstructive sleep apnea syndrome: a study based on computerized measures. Brain Cogn 2017;117:26–32.

18. Kilpinen R, Saunamäki T, Jehkonen M. Information processing speed in obstructive sleep apnea syndrome: a review. Acta Neurol Scand 2014;129(4): 209–18.

19. Ferini-Strambi L, Baietto C, Di Gioia MR, et al. Cognitive dysfunction in patients with obstructive sleep apnea (OSA): partial reversibility after continuous positive airway pressure (CPAP). Brain Res Bull 2003;61(1):87–92.

20. Khassawneh BY, Bathgate CJ, Tsai SC, et al. Neurocognitive performance in insomnia disorder: the impact of hyperarousal and short sleep duration. J Sleep Res 2018;27(6):e12747.

21. Yaouhi K, Bertran F, Clochon P, et al. A combined neuropsychological and brain imaging study of obstructive sleep apnea. J Sleep Res 2009;18(1): 36–48.

22. Aloia MS, Arnedt JT, Davis JD, et al. Neuropsychological sequelae of obstructive sleep apnea-hypopnea syndrome: a critical review. Journal of the International Neuropsychological Society 2004; 10(5):772–85.

23. Vignola A, Lamoureux C, Bastien CH, et al. Effects of chronic insomnia and use of benzodiazepines on daytime performance in older adults. J Gerontol Ser B 2000;55(1):P54–62.

24. Rouleau I, Décary A, Chicoine A-J, et al. Procedural skill learning in obstructive sleep apnea syndrome. Sleep 2002;25(4):398–408.

25. Mathieu A, Mazza S, Décary A, et al. Effects of obstructive sleep apnea on cognitive function: a comparison between younger and older OSAS patients. Sleep Med 2008;9(2):112–20.

26. Neu D, Kajosch H, Peigneux P, et al. Cognitive impairment in fatigue and sleepiness associated conditions. Psychiatry Res 2011;189(1):128–34.

27. Landry S, Anderson C, Andrewartha P, et al. The impact of obstructive sleep apnea on motor skill

acquisition and consolidation. J Clin Sleep Med 2014;10(5):491–6.

28. Causby R, Reed L, McDonnell M, et al. Use of objective psychomotor tests in health professionals. Percept Mot Skills 2014;118(3):765–804.

29. Ayalon RD, Friedman F. The effect of sleep deprivation on fine motor coordination in obstetrics and gynecology residents. Am J Obstet Gynecol 2008; 199(5):576.e1-5.

30. Bawden FC, Oliveira CA, Caramelli P. Impact of obstructive sleep apnea on cognitive performance. Arq Neuropsiquiatr 2011;69(4):585–9.

31. Saunamäki T, Himanen S-L, Polo O, et al. Executive dysfunction and learning effect after continuous positive airway pressure treatment in patients with obstructive sleep apnea syndrome. Eur Neurol 2010;63(4):215–20.

32. Verstraeten E, Cluydts R, Pevernagie D, et al. Executive function in sleep apnea: controlling for attentional capacity in assessing executive attention. Sleep 2004;27(4):685–93.

33. Saunamäki T, Himanen S-L, Polo O, et al. Executive dysfunction in patients with obstructive sleep apnea syndrome. Eur Neurol 2009;62(4):237–42.

34. Twigg GL, Papaioannou I, Jackson M, et al. Obstructive sleep apnea syndrome is associated with deficits in verbal but not visual memory. Am J Respir Crit Care Med 2010;182(1):98–103.

35. Van Dongen HPA, Maislin G, Mullington JM, et al. The cumulative cost of additional wakefulness: dose-response effects on neurobehavioral functions and sleep physiology from chronic sleep restriction and total sleep deprivation. Sleep 2003; 26(2):117–26.

36. Vance DE, Heaton K, Fazeli PL, et al. Aging, speed of processing training, and everyday functioning: implications for practice and research. Activities, Adaptation & Aging 2010;34(4):276–91.

37. Ebaid D, Crewther SG, MacCalman K, et al. Cognitive processing speed across the lifespan: beyond the influence of motor speed. Front Aging Neurosci 2017;9:62.

38. Beebe DW, Groesz L, Wells C, et al. The neuropsychological effects of obstructive sleep apnea: a meta-analysis of norm-referenced and case-controlled data. Sleep 2003;26(3):298–307.

39. Olaithe M, Bucks RS. Executive dysfunction in OSA before and after treatment: a meta-analysis. Sleep 2013;36(9):1297–305.

40. Gagnon K, Baril A-A, Gagnon J-F, et al. Cognitive impairment in obstructive sleep apnea. Pathol Biol (Paris) 2014;62(5):233–40.

41. Ballard JC. Computerized assessment of sustained attention: a review of factors affecting vigilance performance. J Clin Exp Neuropsychol 1996; 18(6):843–63.

42. Basner M, Dinges DF. Maximizing sensitivity of the Psychomotor Vigilance Test (PVT) to sleep loss. Sleep 2011;34(5):581–91.

43. Batool-Anwar S, Kales SN, Patel SR, et al. Obstructive sleep apnea and psychomotor vigilance task performance. Nat Sci Sleep 2014;6:65–71.

44. Huang Y, Hennig S, Fietze I, et al. The Psychomotor Vigilance Test compared to a divided attention steering simulation in patients with moderate or severe obstructive sleep apnea. Nat Sci Sleep 2020; 12:509–24.

45. Li N, Wang J, Wang D, et al. Correlation of sleep microstructure with daytime sleepiness and cognitive function in young and middle-aged adults with obstructive sleep apnea syndrome. Eur Arch Otorhinolaryngol 2019;276(12):3525–32.

46. Djonlagic I, Guo M, Igue M, et al. REM-related obstructive sleep apnea: when does it matter? Effect on motor memory consolidation versus emotional health. J Clin Sleep Med 2020;16(3): 377–84.

47. Sforza E, Haba-Rubio J, De Bilbao F, et al. Performance vigilance task and sleepiness in patients with sleep-disordered breathing. Eur Respir J 2004;24(2):279–85.

48. Kim H, Suh S, Cho ER, et al. Longitudinal course of insomnia: age-related differences in subjective sleepiness and vigilance performance in a population-based sample. J Psychosom Res 2013;75(6):532–8.

49. Hansen DA, Layton ME, Riedy SM, et al. Psychomotor vigilance impairment during total sleep deprivation is exacerbated in sleep-onset insomnia. Nat Sci Sleep 2019;11:401–10.

50. Altena E, Van Der Werf YD, Strijers RLM, et al. Sleep loss affects vigilance: effects of chronic insomnia and sleep therapy. J Sleep Res 2008; 17(3):335–43.

51. Edinger JD, Glenn DM, Bastian LA, et al. Slow-wave sleep and waking cognitive performance II: findings among middle-aged adults with and without insomnia complaints. Physiol Behav 2000; 70(1–2):127–34.

52. Perrier J, Chavoix C, Bocca ML. Functioning of the three attentional networks and vigilance in primary insomnia. Sleep Med 2015;16(12):1569–75.

53. Shekleton JA, Flynn-Evans EE, Miller B, et al. Neurobehavioral performance impairment in insomnia: relationships with self-reported sleep and daytime functioning. Sleep 2014;37(1):107–16.

54. Dorrian J, Rogers NL, Dinges DF. Psychomotor vigilance performance: a neurocognitive assay sensitive to sleep loss. In: Kushida C, editor. Sleep Deprivation: Clinical Issues, Pharmacology and Sleep Loss Effects. New York: Marcel Dekker; 2005. p. 39–70.

55. Basner M, Mollicone D, Dinges DF. Validity and sensitivity of a brief Psychomotor Vigilance Test (PVT-B) to total and partial sleep deprivation. Acta Astronaut 2011;69(11–12):949–59.

56. Benderoth S, Hörmann HJ, Schießl C, et al. Reliability and validity of a 3-minute psychomotor vigilance task (PVT) in assessing sensitivity to sleep loss and alcohol: fitness for duty in aviation and transportation. Sleep 2021. https://doi.org/10.1093/sleep/zsab151.

57. Woods H, Marchetti LM, Biello SM, et al. The clock as a focus of selective attention in those with primary insomnia: an experimental study using a modified Posner paradigm. Behav Res Ther 2009;47(3):231–6.

58. Jones BT, Macphee LM, Broomfield NM, et al. Sleep-related attentional bias in good, moderate, and poor (primary insomnia) sleepers. J Abnorm Psychol 2005;114(2):249–58.

59. Marchetti LM, Biello SM, Broomfield NM, et al. Who is pre-occupied with sleep? A comparison of attention bias in people with psychophysiological insomnia, delayed sleep phase syndrome and good sleepers using the induced change blindness paradigm. J Sleep Res 2006;15(2):212–21.

60. Wermes R, Lincoln TM, Helbig-Lang S. How well can we measure visual attention? Psychometric properties of manual response times and first fixation latencies in a visual search paradigm. Cogn Ther Res 2017;41(4):588–99.

61. Miyake A, Friedman NP, Emerson MJ, et al. The unity and diversity of executive functions and their contributions to complex "Frontal Lobe" tasks: a latent variable analysis. Cogn Psychol 2000;41(1):49–100.

62. Lehto JE, Juujärvi P, Kooistra L, et al. Dimensions of executive functioning: evidence from children. Br J Dev Psychol 2003;21(1):59–80. https://doi.org/10.1348/026151003321164627.

63. Diamond A. Executive functions. Annu Rev Psychol 2013;64:135–68.

64. Ballesio A, Aquino MRJV, Kyle SD, et al. Executive functions in insomnia disorder: a systematic review and exploratory meta-analysis. Front Psychol 2019;10:101.

65. Saunamäki T, Jehkonen M. A review of executive functions in obstructive sleep apnea syndrome. Acta Neurol Scand 2007;115(1):1–11.

66. Fortier-Brochu E, Beaulieu-Bonneau S, Ivers H, et al. Insomnia and daytime cognitive performance: a meta-analysis. Sleep Med Rev 2012;16(1):83–94.

67. Wechsler D. WAiS-Iii. San Antonio: Psychological Corporation; 1997.

68. Kirchner WK. Age differences in short-term retention of rapidly changing information. J Exp Psychol 1958;55(4):352–8.

69. Aasvik J, Stiles TC, Woodhouse A, et al. The effect of insomnia on neuropsychological functioning in patients with comorbid symptoms of pain, fatigue, and mood disorders. Arch Clin Neuropsychol 2018;33(1):14–23.

70. Torelli F, Moscufo N, Garreffa G, et al. Cognitive profile and brain morphological changes in obstructive sleep apnea. Neuroimage 2011;54(2):787–93.

71. Werli KS, Otuyama LJ, Bertolucci PH, et al. Neurocognitive function in patients with residual excessive sleepiness from obstructive sleep apnea: a prospective, controlled study. Sleep Med 2016;26:6–11.

72. Canessa N, Castronovo V, Cappa SF, et al. Sleep apnea: altered brain connectivity underlying a working-memory challenge. Neuroimage Clin 2018;19:56–65.

73. Thomas RJ, Rosen BR, Stern CE, et al. Functional imaging of working memory in obstructive sleep-disordered breathing. J Appl Physiol (1985) 2005;98(6):2226–34.

74. Naëgelé B, Launois SH, Mazza S, et al. Which memory processes are affected in patients with obstructive sleep apnea? An evaluation of 3 types of memory. Sleep 2006;29(4):533–44.

75. Haimov I, Hanuka E, Horowitz Y. Chronic insomnia and cognitive functioning among older adults. Behav Sleep Med 2008;6(1):32–54.

76. Cellini N, de Zambotti M, Covassin N, et al. Working memory impairment and cardiovascular hyperarousal in young primary insomniacs. Psychophysiology 2014;51(2):206–14.

77. Lovato N, Lack L, Wright H, et al. Working memory performance of older adults with insomnia. J Sleep Res 2013;22(3):251–7.

78. Hommel B. Inverting the Simon effect by intention. Psychol Res 1993;55(4):270–9.

79. Eriksen CW. The flankers task and response competition: a useful tool for investigating a variety of cognitive problems. Vis Cogn 1995;2(2–3):101–18.

80. Williams BJ, Kaufmann LM. Reliability of the go/No go association task. J Exp Social Psychol 2012;48(4):879–91.

81. Congdon E, Mumford JA, Cohen JR, et al. Measurement and reliability of response inhibition. Front Psychol 2012;3:37.

82. Tulek B, Atalay NB, Kanat F, et al. Attentional control is partially impaired in obstructive sleep apnea syndrome. J Sleep Res 2013;22(4):422–9.

83. Cross NE, Carrier J, Postuma RB, et al. Association between insomnia disorder and cognitive function in middle-aged and older adults: a cross-sectional analysis of the Canadian Longitudinal Study on Aging. Sleep 2019;42(8). https://doi.org/10.1093/sleep/zsz114.

84. Sivertsen B, Hysing M, Wehling E, et al. Neuropsychological performance in older insomniacs. Neuropsychol Dev Cogn B Aging Neuropsychol Cogn 2013;20(1):34–48.

85. Pearson VE, Allen RP, Dean T, et al. Cognitive deficits associated with restless legs syndrome (RLS). Sleep Med 2006;7(1):25–30.

86. Covassin N, de Zambotti M, Sarlo M, et al. Cognitive performance and cardiovascular markers of hyperarousal in primary insomnia. Int J Psychophysiol 2011;80(1):79–86.

87. Sagaspe P, Philip P, Schwartz S. Inhibitory motor control in apneic and insomniac patients: a stop task study. J Sleep Res 2007;16(4):381–7.

88. Zhao W, Gao D, Yue F, et al. Response inhibition deficits in insomnia disorder: an event-related potential study with the stop-signal task. Front Neurol 2018;9:610.

89. Angelelli P, Macchitella L, Toraldo DM, et al. The neuropsychological profile of attention deficits of patients with obstructive sleep apnea: an update on the daytime attentional impairment. Brain Sci 2020;10(6).

90. Salorio CF, White DA, Piccirillo J, et al. Learning, memory, and executive control in individuals with obstructive sleep apnea syndrome. J Clin Exp Neuropsychol 2002;24(1):93–100.

91. de Almondes KM, Júnior FWNH, Leonardo MEM, et al. Facial emotion recognition and executive functions in insomnia disorder: an exploratory study. Front Psychol 2020;11:502.

92. Fang S-C, Huang C-J, Yang T-T, et al. Heart rate variability and daytime functioning in insomniacs and normal sleepers: preliminary results. J Psychosom Res 2008;65(1):23–30.

93. Ju G, Yoon I-Y, Lee SD, et al. Effects of sleep apnea syndrome on delayed memory and executive function in elderly adults. J Am Geriatr Soc 2012;60(6):1099–103.

94. Delazer M, Zamarian L, Frauscher B, et al. Oxygen desaturation during night sleep affects decision-making in patients with obstructive sleep apnea. J Sleep Res 2016;25(4):395–403.

95. Rist PM, Elbaz A, Dufouil C, et al. Restless legs syndrome and cognitive function: a population-based cross-sectional study. Am J Med 2015;128(9):1023.e3-9.

96. Sdoia S, Ferlazzo F. Stimulus-related inhibition of task set during task switching. Exp Psychol 2008;55(5):322–7.

97. Wilckens KA, Hall MH, Erickson KI, et al. Task switching in older adults with and without insomnia. Sleep Med 2017;30:113–20.

98. Ballesio A, Cerolini S, Ferlazzo F, et al. The effects of one night of partial sleep deprivation on executive functions in individuals reporting chronic insomnia and good sleepers. J Behav Ther Exp Psychiatry 2018;60:42–5.

99. Baldo JV, Shimamura AP, Delis DC, et al. Verbal and design fluency in patients with frontal lobe lesions. J Int Neuropsychol Soc 2001;7(5):586–96.

100. Moscovitch M, Cabeza R, Winocur G, et al. Episodic memory and beyond: the Hippocampus and Neocortex in transformation. Annu Rev Psychol 2016;67:105–34.

101. Lezak MD, Howieson DB, Bigler ED, et al. Neuropsychological assessment. 5th edition. New York: Oxford University Press; 2012.

102. Wallace A, Bucks RS. Memory and obstructive sleep apnea: a meta-analysis. Sleep 2013;36(2):203–20.

103. Cosentino FII, Bosco P, Drago V, et al. The APOE epsilon4 allele increases the risk of impaired spatial working memory in obstructive sleep apnea. Sleep Med 2008;9(8):831–9.

104. Gale SD, Hopkins RO. Effects of hypoxia on the brain: neuroimaging and neuropsychological findings following carbon monoxide poisoning and obstructive sleep apnea. J Int Neuropsychol Soc 2004;10(1):60–71.

105. Ayalon L, Ancoli-Israel S, Klemfuss Z, et al. Increased brain activation during verbal learning in obstructive sleep apnea. Neuroimage 2006;31(4):1817–25.

106. Adams N, Strauss M, Schluchter M, et al. Relation of measures of sleep-disordered breathing to neuropsychological functioning. Am J Respir Crit Care Med 2001;163(7):1626–31.

107. Prigatano GP. Wechsler Memory Scale: a selective review of the literature. J Clin Psychol 1978;34(4):816–32.

108. Daurat A, Foret J, Bret-Dibat J-L, et al. Spatial and temporal memories are affected by sleep fragmentation in obstructive sleep apnea syndrome. J Clin Exp Neuropsychol 2008;30(1):91–101.

109. Killgore WDS, Kendall AP, Richards JM, et al. Lack of degradation in visuospatial perception of line orientation after one night of sleep loss. Percept Mot Skills 2007;105(1):276–86.

110. Venkatraman V, Chuah YML, Huettel SA, et al. Sleep deprivation elevates expectation of gains and attenuates response to losses following risky decisions. Sleep 2007;30(5):603–9.

111. Bechara A, Damasio H, Damasio AR. Emotion, decision making and the orbitofrontal cortex. Cereb Cortex 2000;10(3):295–307.

112. Daurat A, Ricarrère M, Tiberge M. Decision making is affected in obstructive sleep apnoea syndrome. J Neuropsychol 2013;7(1):139–44.

113. McNally KA, Shear PK, Tlustos S, et al. Iowa gambling task performance in overweight children and adolescents at risk for obstructive sleep apnea. J Int Neuropsychol Soc 2012;18(3):481–9.

114. Chunhua X, Jiacui D, Xue L, et al. Impaired emotional memory and decision-making following

primary insomnia. Medicine (Baltimore) 2019; 98(29):e16512.

115. Bayard S, Yu H, Langenier MC, et al. Decision making in restless legs syndrome. Mov Disord 2010; 25(15):2634–40.

116. Bayard S, Langenier MC, Dauvilliers Y. Decision-making, reward-seeking behaviors and dopamine agonist therapy in restless legs syndrome. Sleep 2013;36(10):1501–7.

117. Lejuez CW, Read JP, Kahler CW, et al. Evaluation of a behavioral measure of risk taking: the balloon analogue risk task (BART). J Exp Psychol Appl 2002;8(2):75–84.

118. Bornovalova MA, Daughters SB, Hernandez GD, et al. Differences in impulsivity and risk-taking propensity between primary users of crack cocaine and primary users of heroin in a residential substance-use program. Exp Clin Psychopharmacol 2005;13(4):311–8.

119. Heinrich EC, Djokic MA, Gilbertson D, et al. Cognitive function and mood at high altitude following acclimatization and use of supplemental oxygen and adaptive servoventilation sleep treatments. PLoS One 2019;14(6):e0217089.

120. Demos KE, Hart CN, Sweet LH, et al. Partial sleep deprivation impacts impulsive action but not impulsive decision-making. Physiol Behav 2016;164(Pt A):214–9.

121. Heim B, Pertl M-T, Stefani A, et al. Haste makes waste: decision making in patients with restless legs syndrome with and without augmentation. PLoS One 2017;12(4):e0174793.

122. Heim B, Pertl M-T, Stefani A, et al. Reflection impulsivity perceptual decision-making in patients with restless legs syndrome. Ann Clin Transl Neurol 2018;5(3):315–22.

123. Djamshidian A, O'Sullivan SS, Sanotsky Y, et al. Decision making, impulsivity, and addictions: do Parkinson's disease patients jump to conclusions? Mov Disord 2012;27(9):1137–45.

124. Furl N, Averbeck BB. Parietal cortex and insula relate to evidence seeking relevant to reward-related decisions. J Neurosci 2011;31(48): 17572–82.

125. Heim B, Ellmerer P, Stefani A, et al. Birds of a feather flock together: disadvantageous decision making in augmented restless legs syndrome patients with and without impulse control disorders. Brain Sci 2021;11(3). https://doi.org/10.3390/brainsci11030383.

126. Daniela T, Alessandro C, Giuseppe C, et al. Lack of sleep affects the evaluation of emotional stimuli. Brain Res Bull 2010;82(1):104–8.

127. Goldstein-Piekarski AN, Greer SM, Saletin JM, et al. Sleep deprivation impairs the human central and peripheral nervous system discrimination of social threat. J Neurosci 2015;35(28):10135–45.

128. Guadagni V, Burles F, Valera S, et al. The relationship between quality of sleep and emotional empathy. J Psychophysiology 2017;31(4):158–66.

129. Bucks RS, Olaithe M, Rosenzweig I, et al. Reviewing the relationship between OSA and cognition: where do we go from here? Respirology 2017; 22(7):1253–61.

130. Stocker RPJ, Khan H, Henry L, et al. Effects of sleep loss on subjective complaints and objective neurocognitive performance as measured by the immediate post-concussion assessment and cognitive testing. Arch Clin Neuropsychol 2017; 32(3):349–68.

131. Wang M-L, Wang C, Tuo M, et al. Cognitive effects of treating obstructive sleep apnea: a meta-analysis of randomized controlled trials. J Alzheimers Dis 2020;75(3):705–15.

132. Aloia MS, Arnedt JT, Davis JD, et al. Neuropsychological sequelae of obstructive sleep apnea-hypopnea syndrome: a critical review. J Int Neuropsychol Soc 2004;10(5):772–85.

133. Décary A, Rouleau I, Montplaisir J. Cognitive deficits associated with sleep apnea syndrome: a proposed neuropsychological test battery. Sleep 2000;23(3):369–81.

134. Feenstra HEM, Vermeulen IE, Murre JMJ, et al. Online cognition: factors facilitating reliable online neuropsychological test results. Clin Neuropsychol 2017;31(1):59–84.

135. KIM J, PARK E, AN M. The cognitive impact of chronic diseases on functional capacity in community-dwelling adults. J Nurs Res 2019; 27(1):1–8.

136. Wennberg AMV, Wu MN, Rosenberg PB, et al. Sleep disturbance, cognitive decline, and dementia: a review. Semin Neurol 2017;37(4):395–406.

137. Siedlecki KL, Tucker-Drob EM, Oishi S, et al. Life satisfaction across adulthood: different determinants at different ages? J Posit Psychol 2008; 3(3):153–64.

138. Basner M, Hermosillo E, Nasrini J, et al. Repeated administration effects on Psychomotor Vigilance Test performance. Sleep 2018;41(1). https://doi.org/10.1093/sleep/zsx187.

139. Deary IJ, Liewald D, Nissan J. A free, easy-to-use, computer-based simple and four-choice reaction time programme: the Deary-Liewald reaction time task. Behav Res 2011;43(1):258–68.

140. Wechsler D. Wechsler adult intelligence scale -Fourth Edition (WAIS -IV). San Antonio: NCS Pearson 2008;22(498):816-27.

141. Hutchison KA, Balota DA, Neely JH, et al. The semantic priming project. Behav Res 2013;45(4): 1099–114.

142. Mioshi E, Dawson K, Mitchell J, et al. The Addenbrooke's Cognitive Examination Revised (ACE-R):

a brief cognitive test battery for dementia screening. Int J Geriatr Psychiatry 2006;21(11):1078–85.

143. Ciesielska N, Sokołowski R, Mazur E, et al. Is the Montreal Cognitive Assessment (MoCA) test better suited than the Mini-Mental State Examination (MMSE) in mild cognitive impairment (MCI) detection among people aged over 60? Meta-analysis. Psychiatr Pol 2016;50(5):1039–52.

144. Wechsler D. Wechsler Abbreviated Scale of Intelligence WASI-II . San Antonio: Manual.; 2011.

145. Ryan JJ, Lopez SJ. Wechsler Adult intelligence scale-III. In: Dorfman WI, Hersen M, editors. *Understanding psychological assessment*. Perspectives on individual differences. New York: Springer US; 2001. p. 19–42. https://doi.org/10.1007/978-1-4615-1185-4_2.

146. Del Rossi G, Malaguti A, Del Rossi S. Practice effects associated with repeated assessment of a clinical test of reaction time. J Athl Train 2014; 49(3):356–9.

The Role of Patient-Reported Outcomes in Sleep Measurements

Dirk Pevernagie, MD, PhD[a,b,]*, Fré A. Bauters, MD, PhD[a,b],
Katrien Hertegonne, MD, PhD[a,b]

KEYWORDS

- Sleep • Sleep medicine • Questionnaire • Patient-reported outcome • Polysomnography

KEY POINTS

- Sleep disorders must be assessed subjectively and objectively.
- Subjective assessment includes the medical interview and administration of dedicated questionnaires or patient-reported outcome measures (PROMs).
- Generic and disease-specific PROMs are available for a variety of sleep disorders.
- PROMs have inherent limitations and future research should aim to improve them.
- PROMs have become increasingly important in clinical research and health outcomes assessments.

INTRODUCTION

Sleep, next to healthy nutrition and exercise, is the third fundamental pillar of good health. Disordered sleep is often associated with decreased health-related quality of life (HRQoL) and may predispose to socioeconomic adversity in many affected subjects.[1] Sleep disorders may constitute distinct medical conditions or may complicate other somatic or psychiatric diseases.[2] Adverse biomedical and psychosocial conditions[3–6] as well as unfavorable socioenvironmental factors[7] negatively affect sleep and may play a significant role in the clinical manifestation of sleep disorders. Owing to lack of education on the physiology and pathology of sleep in the curriculum of health care professionals, these disorders remain often underdiagnosed and, consequently, not well treated.[4,8] The use of questionnaires on sleep and sleep disorders may help the practitioner to compensate for this knowledge gap. Moreover, assessment of disordered sleep by applying structured enquiries may be instrumental for making suitable differential diagnosis and offering patient-centered care.

Sleep disorders are assessed the same way as any other medical problem. The history is key to formulating a working hypothesis that may be corroborated (or rejected) by physical examination and targeted technical investigations. To confirm a tentative diagnosis and to assess disease severity, sleep can be measured with different instruments. Polysomnography (PSG) is considered the gold standard for this purpose.[9] PSG is carried out by overnight recording of neurophysiological and cardiorespiratory signals, followed by detailed analysis of the content and finalized by interpretation of the results by a sleep specialist.[10] Thus, the biologic signals of PSG capture adverse events in sleep that compromise its quality. PSG is a reliable instrument for the objective assessment and quantification of sleep-related pathophysiological phenomena.

Surprisingly, in many patients, no robust correlation can be demonstrated between the "pathophysiological severity" of the disorder as

[a] Department of Respiratory Medicine, Ghent University Hospital, Gent, Corneel Heymanslaan 10, Gent 9000, Belgium; [b] Department of Internal Medicine and Paediatrics, Faculty of Medicine and Health Sciences, Ghent University, Corneel Heymanslaan 10, Gent 9000, Belgium
* Corresponding author.
E-mail address: dirk.pevernagie@ugent.be

Sleep Med Clin 16 (2021) 595–606
https://doi.org/10.1016/j.jsmc.2021.07.001
1556-407X/21/© 2021 The Authors. Published by Elsevier Inc. This is an open access article under the CC BY-NC-ND license (http://creativecommons.org/licenses/by-nc-nd/4.0/).

evidenced by markers on PSG and the "clinical severity" as indicated by the seriousness of symptoms and signs. Especially, the lack of association between the apnea-hypopnea index (AHI), a polysomnographic marker of severity in obstructive sleep apnea (OSA), and clinical manifestations of this condition has become evident in recent years.[11] Studies appraising associations between AHI and indices of HRQoL have also failed to demonstrate any significant relationships.[12–14] Such lack of correspondence may indicate that the pathophysiology-driven model of sleep-disordered breathing does not satisfactorily capture disease heterogeneity and does not identify the subtleties that constitute the individual's clinical picture. This lack of correspondence may hold true for nonrespiratory sleep disorders as well. The AHI and potentially other biomarkers emanating from pathophysiological paradigms may have insufficient power to predict clinical relevance and their use as surrogate markers for disease severity may be misleading.[11] In sleep medicine, as in other disciplines, it is mandatory to apply a broad range of examinations for establishing a correct diagnosis and for rating disease severity. In this respect, the medical interview still is the cornerstone of the clinical workup.

Treatment is primarily aimed to remedy the underlying cause of the diagnosed sleep disorder. In OSA, for example, the therapeutic goal is to lower the AHI by preventing passive collapse of the upper airway during sleep. Normalization of the AHI, however, is not always associated with sufficient improvement of daytime symptoms (**Box 1**).[15] In this case, alternative diagnoses or associated comorbidities must be further explored. Thus, restoration of the physiologic process is not an exclusive proxy for therapeutic success. Systematic reassessment of presenting symptoms is essential and questionnaires that gauge the patient's perceived alterations in symptoms and HRQoL may be used for that purpose.[16] Eventually, the patient's appreciation of her or his own health condition is what matters most.

The patient-reported outcome is instrumental in determining treatment success. A patient-reported outcome measure (PROM) is a questionnaire consisting of several patient-reported outcomes, designed to evaluate symptoms, functioning, and other attributes inherent to HRQoL. Such measures can be developed to assess the outcomes of a certain disease (disease-specific PROMs) or several diseases irrespective of their causes (generic PROMs). PROMs are used in combination with clinical outcome measures (COMs) to define overall therapeutic success.[17]

> **Box 1**
> **Attribution bias**
>
> A 53-year-old obese male patient presents with complaints of loud snoring and breathing stoppage observed by the bed partner. He reports excessive daytime sleepiness (EDS), as he is unable to remain awake during staff meetings and driving. The AHI, assessed by PSG, is 35/h. The patient is compliant with prescribed CPAP therapy and reports that his snoring is well controlled, much to the satisfaction of his bed partner. His sleepiness, however, is not improved at all. A new PSG under CPAP therapy demonstrates a residual AHI of 2/h and a total sleep time of 674 minutes. An annex MSLT shows a mean sleep latency of 5 minutes, without any REM sleep in the 5 naps. Repeat history taking is remarkable for the persistence of EDS and the need to sleep more than 10 hours per night ever since his early teens. A diagnosis of "idiopathic hypersomnia with long sleep time" is established and treatment with methylphenidate 10 mg t.i.d. is commenced in addition to the already installed CPAP therapy.
>
> This case is remarkable for a spurious association between pathophysiologically relevant sleep-disordered breathing (with an AHI indicative of "severe OSA") and EDS. In this example, the hypersomnolence was primarily caused by an unrelated disorder of the central nervous system.

In this article, we will review the purposes of sleep questionnaires that are used as structured PROMs. Also, we will expand on the multiple purposes of PROMs, on their relevance for value-based health care, and on the necessity to establish standards for appraising the quality of these instruments. Conventional and special approaches to querying patients will be discussed, as well as inherent limitations and opportunities for future developments.

PATIENT-REPORTED OUTCOME MEASURES CAN BE USED FOR DIFFERENT PURPOSES

As a means of structured history taking, questionnaires have been introduced long ago in medical research. PROMs were initially developed for clinical trials, in which they were used to identify eligible participants, to monitor therapeutic efficacy, side effects, and safety of new medical products, and, eventually, to estimate their risk versus benefit ratios.[18] Currently, the use of PROMs has become mandatory in pharmaceutical research.[19]

In clinical practice, PROMs may have different purposes and may serve multiple goals. Screening questionnaires are typically administered in a preclinical phase and are designed to establish the a priori likelihood of a certain diagnosis. Systematic reviews have been published on questionnaires that intend to screen for multiple sleep disorders,[20] and for single diseases such as OSA.[21,22] Further discussion of this matter is outside the scope of this review.

PROMS are especially useful for estimating the relative importance of different symptoms associated with a given clinical condition. Not all complaints are equally troublesome and gathering inclusive information on the different symptoms enables the practitioner to focus on details that matter most to the individual patient.[23] The characteristics of particular traits may provide actionable information suitable for personalized treatment.[24] Likewise, the PROMs that allow for this differentiation should be sensitive enough to monitor effects of treatment and to verify that therapeutic results correspond with the patient's expectations in terms of improvement of HRQoL.[25]

HRQoL can be concisely defined as "the personal health status of an individual."[26,27] Of note, symptom severity may compromise perceived health, but it is not per se synonymous with a decreased quality of life. Actually, HRQoL is a multiple domain concept not only referring to experiences of illness such as pain, fatigue, and disability but also considering broader aspects of the individual's physical, emotional, and social wellbeing.[16] Different constructs of HRQoL exist, but when used in a research domain, the chosen model should be consistently applied.[28]

PROMs are increasingly used to standardize medical practice and to assess the effectiveness of organized health care. Research on patient-centered outcomes makes use of aggregated PROMs data to compare the effectiveness of different providers with the aim to support quality improvement in health care.[29] Value-based health care is a prevailing health-economical model in which COMs and PROMs are combined into standard sets for appraising treatment outcomes of various diseases.[30] As outcomes are based on patients' priorities, the role of internationally validated, high-quality PROMs is paramount in the assessment strategy of value-based health care.[17] From an integrative perspective, there is a case for pooling the intentions and efforts of the various stakeholders (ie, clinicians, patients, researchers, and health care insurers) to endorse sustainable data collection systems in which PROMs are administered at intake and in the course of treatment. Such comprehensive approach is expected to stimulate meaningful use in research, clinical practice, and quality improvement programs.[31]

QUALITY AND REPORTING OF PATIENT-REPORTED OUTCOME MEASURES

Measurement properties of PROMs must comply with rigorous standards as shown in **Table 1**. The quality prerequisites of a PROM must be tested before release for large-scale use. Recommendations regarding the design and implementation of new questionnaires are available in the literature.[32–35] Also, there are guidelines on how to assess the methodological quality of existing PROMs.[36] The International Society for Quality of Life Research (ISOQOL) has published a set of standards itemizing different properties that a PROM should be tested for (see **Table 1**).[37] Together, these properties define the "validity," being the agreement between what a PROM actually measures in view of what it purports to measure. The role of patients is very important in determining the content aspect of validity—the target population should be involved already in the initial phase of designing a new PROM. Finally, PROMs should not be regarded as static instruments but should be updated in the course of time with the aim of improving their measurement properties in a "PROM cycle."[35]

As already mentioned, PROMs consist of separate questions that may be grouped into different domains reflecting various dimensions of a certain disease. To determine the dimensionality of a PROM in terms of different symptoms or HRQoL aspects, items can be grouped together based on the clinical relevance of symptoms. This is called a "clinimetric" method. In contrast, the application of principal component analysis (ie, statistical analysis of items in a covariant matrix) is known as a "psychometric" approach.[38,39] Both methods can be used to decide on the content of a PROM. The questions themselves test the severity of a phenomenon (a symptom, generally speaking) in terms of intensity and frequency over time. Furthermore, it can be appraised to what extent various symptoms pose a problem regarding different aspects of HRQoL. Usually, the results of the separate items are computed into scores per domain and/or a global score reflecting the overall subjective severity of the disease. Moreover, several options exist to visualize the results of PROMs. **Fig. 1** shows an overview of common graphical illustrations of symptoms and domains.

PATIENT-REPORTED OUTCOME MEASURES IN SLEEP MEDICINE

Since the 1990s, several PROMs have been introduced for different purposes in the field of sleep

Table 1
Definition of PROM properties

Conceptual and measurement model	The conceptual model provides a description and framework for the targeted construct(s) to be included in a PRO measure. The measurement model maps the individual items in the PRO measure to the construct
Reliability	The degree to which a PRO measure is free from measurement error
Internal consistency	The degree of the interrelatedness among the items in a multi-item PRO measure
Test–retest reliability	A measure of the reproducibility of the scale, that is, the ability to provide consistent scores over time in a stable population
Validity	The degree to which a PRO instrument measures the PRO concept it purports to measure
Content validity	The extent to which the PRO measure includes the most relevant and important aspects of a concept in the context of a given measurement application
Construct validity	The degree to which scores on the PRO measure relate to other measures (eg, patient-reported or clinical indicators) in a manner that is consistent with theoretically derived a priori hypotheses concerning the concepts that are being measured
Criterion validity	The degree to which the scores of a PRO measure are an adequate reflection of a "gold standard."
Responsiveness	The extent to which a PRO measure can detect changes in the construct being measured over time
Interpretability of scores	The degree to which one can assign easily understood meaning to a PRO measure's scores
Minimal important difference	Minimal important difference—The smallest difference in score in the outcome of interest that informed patients or informed proxies perceive as important, either beneficial or harmful, and that would lead the patient or clinician to consider a change in the management
Burden	The time, effort, and other demands placed on those to whom the instrument is administered (respondent burden) or on those who administer the instrument (investigator or administrative burden)

Adapted from Reeve et al.[37] with permission from the publisher.

medicine. A distinction is being made between generic questionnaires that may be used in various medical disciplines versus disease-specific questionnaires, designed to gauge symptom severity and HRQoL effects for particular sleep disorders. With respect to disease-specific aspects of sleep medicine, we review frequently used questionnaires in the domains of OSA, insomnia, and restless legs syndrome (RLS).

Generic Questionnaires

Generic questionnaires such as the Medical Outcomes Study 36-item Short Form Health Survey (SF-36)[40] and the EuroQol 5 Dimensions Questionnaire (EQ-5D),[41] among others, have been used to assess HRQoL in patients with sleep disorders. As this target population was not specifically envisaged when these questionnaires were designed, there is little evidence regarding content and other features of measurement validity.[42] The relevance of generic HRQoL instruments for sleep medicine practice is limited and will not be discussed further in this article.

Generic Sleep- and Sleepiness-Related Questionnaires

Two sleep questionnaires, the Pittsburgh Sleep Quality Index (PSQI)[43] and the Epworth Sleepiness

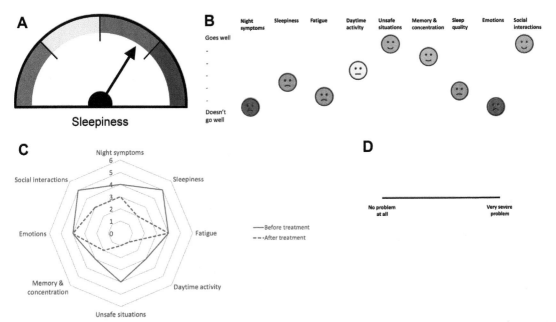

Fig. 1. Different graphical presentations of results from PROMs. (*A*) Graphical presentation of a trait, for example, sleepiness, as a value on a tachometer scale. (*B*) Presentation of different traits on a 7-point Likert scale in parallel columns, using smileys to enhance the visual effect; adapted from Abma and colleagues[39] with permission from the publisher. (*C*) Radar plot with positioning of different traits on a 7-point Likert scale, also showing treatment effects. (*D*) A 1-dimensional visual analog scale.

Scale (ESS),[44] are broadly used in different areas of sleep medicine. The PSQI is suitable for assessing sleep quality in sleep disorders as well as disturbed sleep in other conditions such as mood disorders or pain syndromes.[45] The PSQI consists of 19 questions on a 4-point Likert scale (0–3) and covers 7 domains: subjective sleep quality, sleep latency, sleep duration, sleep efficiency, sleep disturbance, use of hypnotics, and daytime dysfunction. The global score is the sum of all domain items and ranges from 0 to 21. The cutoff for abnormal sleep is >5, with worse sleep quality being associated with higher scores. A review and meta-analysis of the suitability of the PSQI for assessing sleep dysfunction in clinical and nonclinical populations has been published elsewhere.[46] According to this structured review, the PSQI shows strong reliability and validity, and moderate structural validity in a variety of samples, suggesting the tool fulfills its intended utility.

The ESS is a concise PROM composed of 8 questions on a 4-point Likert scale (0–3), yielding scores between 0 and 24, 11 and higher indicating excessive daytime sleepiness. The ESS was originally designed to assess subjective sleepiness in both normal subjects and patients with various sleep disorders.[44] In a separate study on measurement properties, adequate validity was demonstrated for this scale, based on which it was

proposed as a reliable method for measuring daytime sleepiness in adults.[47] However, subsequent studies have shown limited internal consistency, rendering the ESS probably suitable for group but not for individual-level comparisons.[48] The reliability of the ESS in clinical settings is still unproven[49] and its unconditional application has been criticized.[50] Finally, the ESS seems to embody sleepiness better in men than in women who less often have a total score of 11 or higher, although they report feelings of sleepiness as often as men.[51,52]

Patient-Reported Outcome Measures for Obstructive Sleep Apnea

A whole array of questionnaires is currently available for use in OSA. Below, we only report on PROMs that have been subject to appropriate quality assessment and for which measurement properties have been reported.[42] These PROMs are listed in **Table 2**.

The Functional Outcomes of Sleep Questionnaire (FOSQ) is a PROM designed to assess HRQoL in adults suffering from excessive daytime sleepiness. It has been used for studying the effects of treatment with positive airway pressure in OSA patients.[53] The instrument comprises 30-items on a 4-point Likert scale assessing effects

Table 2
Validated PROMs in OSA

Questionnaire	Authors	Content	# Items	# Domains	Likert Scale	Direction
Functional Outcomes of Sleep Questionnaire (FOSQ)	Weaver et al,[54] 1997	Assessing the degree of difficulty for doing activities due to fatigue or being sleepy	30	5	4	↑
OSA Patient-Oriented Severity Index (OSAPOSI)	Piccirillo et al,[55] 1998	Magnitude and importance of problems related to impaired activities, feelings, situations, and behaviors	32	5	6	↓
Calgary Sleep Apnea Quality of Life Index (SAQLI)	Flemons et al,[56] 1998	The disease-related part of the questionnaire probes the amount of time, the amount of difficulty, or the severity associated with certain problems related to activities and functions	56	4	7	↑
Calgary Sleep Apnea Quality of Life Index (SAQLI)	Flemons et al,[56] 1998	The treatment-related part of the questionnaire probes side effects of CPAP therapy in terms of experienced problems	28	N/A	7	↑
Quebec Sleep Questionnaire (QSQ)	Lacasse et al,[57] 2004	Assessing the degree of problems related to impaired activities, feelings, situations, and behaviors	32	5	7	↑
Visual analogical well-being scale (VAWS)	Masa et al,[14] 2011	Rating the degree of the present well-being status between least favorable and most favorable by putting a marker on a horizontal line	1	1	N/A	→
Patient-Reported Apnea Questionnaire (PRAQ)	Abma et al,[39,59,60] 2017–2019	Rating the degree experiencing problems with activities, feelings, situations, and behaviors	40	10	7	↑

Abbreviations: ↑, Higher values indicate a better status; ↓, Higher values indicate a worse status; →, Value to the right indicates a better status; N/A, not available.

of being sleepy or tired on functional performance in 5 domains of health (activity level, general productivity, vigilance, intimate relationships, and social outcome).[54] A global score between 5 and 20 is obtained by computation of the subscales of the 5 domains, a lower score indicating worse HRQoL.

The OSA Patient-Oriented Severity Index (OSA-POSI) consists of 32 questions probing problems in 5 domains (nocturnal sleep, daytime functioning, emotions, productivity, and need of medical care).[55] Each item is assessed according to the severity of the problem on a 6-point Likert scale and the impact on the HRQoL. Higher values correspond with higher impact.

The Calgary Sleep Apnea Quality of Life Index (SAQLI) comprises 56 disease-related and 28 treatment-related questions.[56] Each item is rated on a 7-point Likert scale. The following domains are covered: daily functioning, social interactions, emotional functioning, and symptoms. Also, unwanted treatment-induced side effects are registered. The questions encompass the amount of time a problem is present, the amount of difficulty a person experiences with a certain problem, or the severity of the problem itself. In contrast with the other OSA questionnaires that can be filled out by the patients themselves, this elaborate PROM was designed to be administered by an interviewer.

The Quebec Sleep Questionnaire (QSQ) lists 32 questions on a 7-point Likert scale, querying the degree of problems associated with daytime sleepiness, diurnal symptoms, nocturnal symptoms, emotions, and social interactions.[57] The mean scores of the 5 domains are computed to produce a total score, positively reflecting HRQoL. The instrument's responsiveness is adequate to show subtle changes induced by treatment. Although the SAQLI and QSQ bear similarities, a notable difference between the two is that the former is based on a "psychometric" factor analysis model, whereas the latter results from a "clinimetric" disease impact approach.[58]

Masa and colleagues[14] developed a PROM for OSA based on a simple visual analogical wellbeing scale (VAWS) and assessed its performance in respect of existing HRQoL questionnaires. VAWS correlated with all HRQoL tests but better with FOSQ and EQ-5D. Furthermore, VAWS and FOSQ correlated better with clinical variables (restlessness and snoring) than other HRQoL tests. VAWS captured effects of treatment similarly to FOSQ but better than other HRQoL tests. VAWS was promoted as a very simple tool for testing HRQoL in OSA before and after treatment.

The OSA-specific questionnaires described earlier have been criticized for incomplete validation and the lack of certainty about measurement error.[42] Recently, a new PROM for OSA has been developed, involving patients in all the consecutive steps of instrument validation. The Patient-Reported Apnea Questionnaire (PRAQ) consists of 40 questions on a 7-point Likert scale, probing the degree of difficulties or problems with OSA-related symptoms over 10 health-related domains.[59] The measurement properties are appropriate and responsiveness to treatment seems adequate.[39] Although patients were generally positive about the usefulness of the PRAQ, health care providers reported minor impact on their practices and did not consider the PROM of great help with regard to improving patient-centeredness.[60]

Patient-Reported Outcome Measures for Insomnia

Although insomnia—the inability to fall asleep or to maintain sleep overnight—is a frequent complaint in many common diseases and sleep disorders, it can be a diagnostic entity in its own right. In the latter case, the term "chronic insomnia disorder" is used.[2] Several PROMs have been developed for this condition. The 2 most frequently applied questionnaires are discussed in this section. The aforementioned PSQI is suitable for assessing insomnia severity and for evaluating effects of treatment.[61] The Insomnia Severity Scale (ISI) is a 7-item questionnaire on a 7-point Likert scale, surveying difficulties with initiating or maintaining sleep and associated adverse daytime consequences. Results range between 0 (no insomnia) and 28 (very severe insomnia). Scores between 8 and 14 are considered sub-threshold insomnia.[62] There is convincing evidence to show that the ISI is a reliable instrument for detecting cases of insomnia in the general population, as well as for assessing treatment responses in clinical patients.[63]

Patient-Reported Outcome Measures for Restless Legs Syndrome

RLS is characterized by unpleasant feelings in the lower limbs, and sometimes also the arms or the trunk. These sensations cause an urge to move and are relieved by movement. The symptoms exacerbate in the evening and may prevent patients from falling asleep and/or cause awakenings.[64] PROMs are available to assess symptom severity and response to treatment.

The Restless Legs Syndrome Quality of Life Questionnaire (RLSQLQ) consists of 18 items that gauge the effects of RLS on the patient's functioning related to work, social and sexual interactions.[65] Ten of the items yield a global quality-of-life score between 0 and 100, a higher value indicating a better outcome. The other 8 questions deal more in depth with work and sexual interest. The RLSQLQ was found to be a reliable instrument for measuring HRQoL in RLS patients.[65]

The International RLS study group (IRLSSG) has developed a 10-question PROM.[66] This scale, the IRLSSG rating scale (IRLS), grades the severity, frequency, and impact on sleep of RLS symptoms, higher values indicating more severe complaints. The IRLS is not conceived as a screening tool and requires a prior diagnosis of RLS to be used properly. With this scale, spontaneous fluctuations in symptom severity and treatment responsiveness can be assessed. The measurement properties of the IRLS are deemed appropriate.[66]

CONTROVERSIES

Although the methodology of measuring PROs by the systematic application of validated questionnaires has greatly improved our management of various sleep disorders, there are also downsides to this approach. The inexpert use of PROMs may lead to pitfalls that must be acknowledged and addressed.

The use of disease-specific questionnaires may be a source of nosologic bias. On the one hand, symptoms of disturbed sleep such as snoring, inability to sleep, and restlessness may be a manifestation of an underlying condition, for example, alcohol abuse, rheumatic pain, and constitutional eczema, respectively. On the other hand, each of these symptoms may be a key feature of a nosologically defined sleep disorder—in this example, OSA, chronic insomnia disorder, and RLS, respectively. How to interpret symptoms, either as elements of a multisymptomatic condition or as main traits defining a particular phenotype, largely depends on the clinical context. In sleep medicine, generic symptoms and "specific" symptom-based disorders are frequently mixed up.

Many questionnaires constructed around specific sleep disorders are a compilation of nonspecific symptoms that may occur in other conditions as well. A set of symptoms attributed to a particular sleep disorder may overlap with other disorders characterized by a different pathophysiological background. Yet, the assignment of a selection of symptom-based questions to a disease-specific PROM, invariably suggests that all items are causally related to the postulated disease, which is obviously not the case. Therefore, inexpert application of disease-specific PROMs may result in spurious diagnoses and, consequently, inefficient treatment (**Box 2**). In extreme situations, PROMs may generate information that potentially could be (ab)used in ways that disadvantage patients or to limit access to medical services.[67]

In contemporary sleep medicine, the diagnosis of nosologically defined sleep disorders is founded on a combination of a clinical presentation and evidence for pathophysiological abnormalities demonstrated by clinical sleep testing. Although both components may coincide or even be discordant, establishing a diagnosis is frequently straightforward and therapy is mostly effective. Not rarely, however, the clinical presentation is complex. Different sleep disorders may co-occur

---

> **Box 2**
> **Nonspecificity of symptoms**
>
> A patient with severe RLS obtains a total score of 25 on the Insomnia Severity Index, composed of the following subscores: (1) difficulty falling asleep—4; (2) difficulty staying asleep—4; (3) problems with waking up too early—2; (4) dissatisfaction with sleep—4; (5) sleep problem noticeable to others—3; (6) worry and distress—4; and (7) interference with daily activities—4.
>
> This test result could be inadvertently labeled as "very severe insomnia disorder." Yet, treatment with cognitive behavioral therapy would be ineffective in this case because RLS is the causative mechanism.

---

or be complicated by other diseases. Insomnia, for instance, is a common complaint in somatic and/or mental diseases. Moreover, insomnia and OSA co-occur in approximately 30% to 40% of cases.[68] Application of PROMs for specific sleep disorders will only partially map these complex conditions and associated HRQoL impairments. Also, patient-centered treatment outcomes will be incompletely assessed.

Nosologically defined sleep disorders may be heterogeneous in clinical presentation. For example, in OSA, at least 3 different phenotypes have been observed, namely patients with excessive daytime sleepiness, disturbed sleep, or minimal symptoms.[69] These subtypes cannot be discriminated by the AHI, as quite similar AHI values were shown across the 3 groups. Obviously, a case mix of different OSA phenotypes must be included in the validation process of PROMs for OSA. If not, the instrument may predispose to assessing the characteristics of only a certain subgroup. Particularly, subjects who participate in PROM research may belong to subclasses that are not representative of the entire target population.[59] As phenotypical heterogeneity of OSA has only recently been demonstrated, and postdates the publication of legacy OSA questionnaires, it is presumed that all these PROMs may suffer from selection bias to some extent. HRQoL assessment with the FOSQ, for example, only assesses effects of fatigue or being sleepy and does not include effects of disturbed nocturnal sleep.

FUTURE DIRECTIONS: THE NEED FOR NEW PATIENT-REPORTED OUTCOME MEASURES

Can we reliably and beneficially use the existing PROMs in clinical and investigative sleep medicine? The answer is positive, if the user is sufficiently aware of the scope, strengths, and limitations of the different available instruments. Yet, the field lacks an easy-to-use tool—like a clinical thermometer—appealing to both patients and practitioners.[60]

Many sleep centers use a collection of different questionnaires, such as PSQI, ISI, ESS, FOSQ, and so forth, yielding excessive, redundant, and sometimes conflicting information, thus burdening doctors and patients. To overcome this exorbitance, several approaches may be envisaged. The first one is to pool items of existing PROMs that are already validated by patient input. Rather than rely on composite scores of the different domains in separate PROMs, the individual questions of the PROMs might be more suitable for alerting a health care professional to the most important problems of an individual patient.[59]

Another method may consist of extracting distinct traits from disease domains that have proven relevant and to disengage them from conventional—yet still putative—disease models. This way, the constellation of symptoms related to disturbed sleep and daytime dysfunction could be reduced to a minimal set of essential features, for example, insomnia, sleepiness, fatigue, bodily discomfort, and so forth. For each distinct feature, a degree of severity and impact on HRQoL can be assessed. Moreover, by making the PROM free of hypothesis as to a tentative medical diagnosis, preconceptions regarding causality—which is inherent to most disease-specific questionnaires—can be obviated. The expected elimination of bias together with opportunities for multipurpose utility would justify the development of a completely new sleep questionnaire.

When symptoms are nonspecific, a priori coupling with diagnostic outcomes may be speculative. In such conditions, a reference benchmark is required to assure certainty about causation. Although PSG may disclose certain pathophysiological markers, it is often uncertain whether pathophysiology and clinical symptoms are causally linked. Thus, PSG may fall short of providing the required benchmark. Therefore, attribution of causality remains elusive in many patients with sleep complaints. Favorable symptomatic response to treatment, for example, therapy with positive airway pressure for OSA, provides additional evidence regarding the relationship between the presenting symptoms and the purported sleep disorder. Diagnostic therapy is a means not only to assess the degree of symptomatic relief but also to suggest causality.[11] It has been emphasized that PROMs should be sufficiently sensitive to detect treatment-induced changes over time.

Because the observed changes may support diagnostic evidence as well, responsiveness inherently reflects disease-specificity.

Finally, PROMs may become outdated as their content usually remains unchanged, whereas medical concepts and treatments will advance over time. To overcome static inertia, dynamic solutions for obtaining patient-reported outcomes have been developed. The Patient-Reported Outcome Measurement Information System (PROMIS) was established in 2004 with funding from the US National Institutes of Health (NIH).[70] In this configuration, patient-reported outcomes related to different diseases are collected and stored in item banks. These databases include large sets of single questions that comprehensively cover various symptom domains. The collection of items is accessible for computer-adaptive test systems that dynamically compose a (variable) set of patient-reported outcomes depending on the patient's characteristics and on the answers given to preceding questions. The aim is to introduce targeted approaches for capturing relevant patient-centric information, whilst reducing the respondent burden. PROMIS sleep disturbance and sleep-related impairments item banks have been created for assessing sleep disorders.[71] Excellent measurement properties were attributed to this PROM, which was considered useful for probing general aspects of sleep and sleep-related impairments in various groups of patients. This development holds promise for creating future patient-centered assessment instruments in the field of sleep medicine.

SUMMARY

As sleep disorders are highly prevalent, many patients seek appropriate medical help for their sleep problems. Although the medical interview is essential for establishing a diagnostic working hypothesis, questionnaires are valuable add-on tools with respect to clinical subtyping, differential diagnosis, identification of comorbidities, and assessing response to treatment. The term "patient-reported outcome measures" (PROMs) is standard for questionnaires that are validated along a spectrum of different measurement properties. PROMs must comply with rigorous psychometric standards and should be evaluated carefully before release. Sleep disorders can be assessed with generic or disease-specific questionnaires. The latter category comprises PROMs for specific sleep disorders such as OSA, insomnia, and RLS, among others. There are certain limitations to the use of PROMs. The composing traits are often nonspecific and overlap among different nosologic entities. Moreover, PROMs may not capture the full spectrum of disease heterogeneity. Therefore, inappropriate use may yield spurious diagnoses and ineffective treatment. Besides the use of disease-specific instruments, the field of sleep medicine may envisage the introduction of domain-specific questionnaires—free from diagnostic preconceptions—targeting traits that are unique to the patient's condition. This observation may open up perspectives for innovative research on still better PROMs.

CLINICS CARE POINTS

- History taking in patients with sleep disorders can be improved by using self-administered PROMs
- The selection of PROMs should comply with the tentative diagnosis obtained from the medical interview
- PROMs that have an optimal balance between amount of information versus respondent burden are to be preferred
- PROMs are a very important instrument to systematically assess effects of treatment
- Inadvertent use of PROMs is discouraged as such approach inevitably produces spurious diagnoses and inadequate treatment

ACKNOWLEDGMENTS

This work has received funding from the European Union's Horizon 2020 research and innovation program under grant agreement no 965417 Sleep Revolution. The authors thank Prof. Dr. Erna Sif Arnardottir for reviewing the article and for providing pertinent suggestions for improvement.

DISCLOSURE

The authors have nothing to disclose.

REFERENCES

1. Fatima Y, Bucks RS, Mamun AA, et al. Sleep trajectories and mediators of poor sleep: findings from the longitudinal analysis of 41,094 participants of the UK Biobank cohort. Sleep Med 2020;76:120–7.
2. AASM. The international classification of sleep disorders. In: Sateia M, editor. Third edition. Darien (IL): American Academy of Sleep Medicine; 2014.
3. Colten HR, Altevogt BM. Sleep disorders and sleep deprivation: an unmet public health problem. Washinton (DC): National Institutes of Health; 2006.
4. Kapur V, Strohl KP, Redline S, et al. Underdiagnosis of sleep apnea syndrome in U.S. communities. Sleep Breath 2002;6(2):49–54.
5. Young T, Shahar E, Nieto FJ, et al. Predictors of sleep-disordered breathing in community-dwelling adults: the sleep heart health study. Arch Intern Med 2002;162(8):893–900.
6. Mai E, Buysse DJ. Insomnia: prevalence, impact, pathogenesis, differential diagnosis, and evaluation. Sleep Med Clin 2008;3(2):167–74.
7. Johnson DA, Billings ME, Hale L. Environmental determinants of insufficient sleep and sleep disorders: implications for population health. Curr Epidemiol Rep 2018;5(2):61–9.
8. Rosen RC, Zozula R, Jahn EG, et al. Low rates of recognition of sleep disorders in primary care: comparison of a community-based versus clinical academic setting. Sleep Med 2001;2(1):47–55.
9. Kapur VK, Auckley DH, Chowdhuri S, et al. Clinical practice guideline for diagnostic testing for adult obstructive sleep apnea: an American academy of sleep medicine clinical practice guideline. J Clin Sleep Med 2017;13(3):479–504.
10. Berry RB, Brooks R, Gamaldo CE, et al. The AASM manual for the scoring of sleep and associated events. Rules, terminology and technical specifications. Version 2.0. Darien (IL): American Academy of Sleep Medicine; 2012.
11. Pevernagie DA, Gnidovec-Strazisar B, Grote L, et al. On the rise and fall of the apnea-hypopnea index: a historical review and critical appraisal. J Sleep Res 2020;29(4):e13066.
12. Sanner BM, Klewer J, Trumm A, et al. Long-term treatment with continuous positive airway pressure improves quality of life in obstructive sleep apnoea syndrome. Eur Respir J 2000;16(1):118–22.
13. Weaver EM, Woodson BT, Steward DL. Polysomnography indexes are discordant with quality of life, symptoms, and reaction times in sleep apnea patients. Otolaryngol Head Neck Surg 2005;132(2): 255–62.
14. Masa JF, Jimenez A, Duran J, et al. Visual analogical well-being scale for sleep apnea patients: validity and responsiveness : a test for clinical practice. Sleep Breath 2011;15(3):549–59.
15. Foster SN, Hansen SL, Scalzitti NJ, et al. Residual excessive daytime sleepiness in patients with obstructive sleep apnea treated with positive airway pressure therapy. Sleep Breath 2020;24(1):143–50.
16. Garratt A, Schmidt L, Mackintosh A, et al. Quality of life measurement: bibliographic study of patient assessed health outcome measures. BMJ 2002; 324(7351):1417.
17. ICHOM. Standard sets - why measure outcome?. International consortium for health outcomes measurement 2020. Available at: https://www.ichom.org/standard-sets/#about-standard-sets.

18. Willke RJ, Burke LB, Erickson P. Measuring treatment impact: a review of patient-reported outcomes and other efficacy endpoints in approved product labels. Control Clin Trials 2004;25(6):535–52.

19. Wiklund I. Assessment of patient-reported outcomes in clinical trials: the example of health-related quality of life. Fundam Clin Pharmacol 2004;18(3):351–63.

20. Klingman KJ, Jungquist CR, Perlis ML. Questionnaires that screen for multiple sleep disorders. Sleep Med Rev 2017;32:37–44.

21. Nagappa M, Liao P, Wong J, et al. Validation of the STOP-bang questionnaire as a screening tool for obstructive sleep apnea among different populations: a systematic review and meta-analysis. PLoS One 2015;10(12):e0143697.

22. Prasad KT, Sehgal IS, Agarwal R, et al. Assessing the likelihood of obstructive sleep apnea: a comparison of nine screening questionnaires. Sleep Breath 2017;21(4):909–17.

23. Greenhalgh J, Dalkin S, Gooding K, et al. Functionality and feedback: a realist synthesis of the collation, interpretation and utilisation of patient-reported outcome measures data to improve patient care. Health Serv Deliv Res 2017;5(2).

24. Di Paolo A, Sarkozy F, Ryll B, et al. Personalized medicine in Europe: not yet personal enough? BMC Health Serv Res 2017;17(1):289.

25. Revicki D, Hays RD, Cella D, et al. Recommended methods for determining responsiveness and minimally important differences for patient-reported outcomes. J Clin Epidemiol 2008;61(2):102–9.

26. Wilson IB, Cleary PD. Linking clinical variables with health-related quality of life. A conceptual model of patient outcomes. JAMA 1995;273(1):59–65.

27. Acquadro C, Berzon R, Dubois D, et al. Incorporating the patient's perspective into drug development and communication: an ad hoc task force report of the Patient-Reported Outcomes (PRO) Harmonization Group meeting at the Food and Drug Administration, February 16, 2001. Value Health 2003;6(5):522–31.

28. Bakas T, McLennon SM, Carpenter JS, et al. Systematic review of health-related quality of life models. Health Qual Life Outcomes 2012;10:134.

29. Black N. Patient reported outcome measures could help transform healthcare. BMJ 2013;346:f167.

30. Porter ME, Lee TH. The big idea. The strategy that will fix health care. Harv Business Rev 2013;91(10):50–70.

31. Van Der Wees PJ, Nijhuis-Van Der Sanden MW, Ayanian JZ, et al. Integrating the use of patient-reported outcomes for both clinical practice and performance measurement: views of experts from 3 countries. Milbank Q 2014;92(4):754–75.

32. Streiner DN. Health measurement scales: a practical guide to their development and use. 4th edition. Oxford, UK: Oxford University Press; 1995.

33. FDA. Patient-reported outcome measures: use in medical product development to support labeling Claims. Silver Spring, Maryland, USA: Food and Drug Administration; 2009.

34. de Vet HCW, Terwee CB, Mokkink LB, et al. Measurement in medicine - a practical guide. New York, USA: Cambridge University Press; 2011.

35. Verkerk E, Verbiest M, van Dulmen S, et al. PROM-cycle (summary in English). National Health Care Institute of The Netherlands; 2018. https://www.zorginzicht.nl/ontwikkeltools/prom-toolbox/prom-cycle-summary-in-english.

36. Terwee CB, Mokkink LB, Knol DL, et al. Rating the methodological quality in systematic reviews of studies on measurement properties: a scoring system for the COSMIN checklist. Qual Life Res 2012;21(4):651–7.

37. Reeve BB, Wyrwich KW, Wu AW, et al. ISOQOL recommends minimum standards for patient-reported outcome measures used in patient-centered outcomes and comparative effectiveness research. Qual Life Res 2013;22(8):1889–905.

38. de Vet HCWT CB, Bouter LM. Clinimetrics and psychometrics: two sides of the same coin. J Clin Epidemiol 2003;56:1146–7.

39. Abma IL, Rovers M, IJff M, et al. Instrument completion and validation of the patient-reported apnea questionnaire (PRAQ). Health Qual Life Outcomes 2018;16(1):158.

40. Ware JE Jr, Sherbourne CD. The MOS 36-item short-form health survey (SF-36). I. Conceptual framework and item selection. Med Care 1992;30(6):473–83.

41. EuroQol_Group. EuroQol–a new facility for the measurement of health-related quality of life. Health Policy 1990;16(3):199–208.

42. Abma IL, van der Wees PJ, Veer V, et al. Measurement properties of patient-reported outcome measures (PROMs) in adults with obstructive sleep apnea (OSA): a systematic review. Sleep Med Rev 2016;28:18–31.

43. Buysse DJ, Reynolds CF 3rd, Monk TH, et al. The Pittsburgh Sleep Quality Index: a new instrument for psychiatric practice and research. Psychiatry Res 1989;28(2):193–213.

44. Johns MW. A new method for measuring daytime sleepiness: the Epworth sleepiness scale. Sleep 1991;14(6):540–5.

45. Osorio CD, Gallinaro AL, Lorenzi-Filho G, et al. Sleep quality in patients with fibromyalgia using the Pittsburgh sleep quality index. J Rheumatol 2006;33(9):1863–5.

46. Mollayeva T, Thurairajah P, Burton K, et al. The Pittsburgh sleep quality index as a screening tool for sleep dysfunction in clinical and non-clinical samples: a systematic review and meta-analysis. Sleep Med Rev 2016;25:52–73.

47. Johns MW. Reliability and factor analysis of the Epworth sleepiness scale. Sleep 1992;15(4):376–81.

48. Kendzerska TB, Smith PM, Brignardello-Petersen R, et al. Evaluation of the measurement properties of the Epworth sleepiness scale: a systematic review. Sleep Med Rev 2014;18(4):321–31.

49. Taylor E, Zeng I, O'Dochartaigh C. The reliability of the Epworth Sleepiness Score in a sleep clinic population. J Sleep Res 2019;28(2):e12687.

50. Omobomi O, Quan SF. A requiem for the clinical use of the Epworth sleepiness scale. J Clin Sleep Med 2018;14(5):711–2.

51. Baldwin CM, Kapur VK, Holberg CJ, et al. Associations between gender and measures of daytime somnolence in the sleep heart health study. Sleep 2004;27(2):305–11.

52. Arnardottir ES, Islind AS, Oskarsdottir M. The future of sleep measurements - a review and perspective. Sleep Med Clin 2021;16(3):447–64.

53. Billings ME, Rosen CL, Auckley D, et al. Psychometric performance and responsiveness of the functional outcomes of sleep questionnaire and sleep apnea quality of life instrument in a randomized trial: the HomePAP study. Sleep 2014;37(12):2017–24.

54. Weaver TE, Laizner AM, Evans LK, et al. An instrument to measure functional status outcomes for disorders of excessive sleepiness. Sleep 1997;20(10):835–43.

55. Piccirillo JF, Gates GA, White DL, et al. Obstructive sleep apnea treatment outcomes pilot study. Otolaryngol Head Neck Surg 1998;118(6):833–44.

56. Flemons WW, Reimer MA. Development of a disease-specific health-related quality of life questionnaire for sleep apnea. Am J Respir Crit Care Med 1998;158(2):494–503.

57. Lacasse Y, Bureau MP, Series F. A new standardised and self-administered quality of life questionnaire specific to obstructive sleep apnoea. Thorax 2004;59(6):494–9.

58. Sheats RD. Health-related quality of life assessment tools and sleep-disordered breathing. J Dental Sleep Med 2016;3(2):49–55.

59. Abma IL, Rovers M, IJff M, et al. The development of a patient-reported outcome measure for patients with obstructive sleep apnea: the Patient-Reported Apnea Questionnaire (PRAQ). J Patient Rep Outcomes 2017;1(1):14.

60. Abma IL, Rovers MM, IJff M, et al. Does the Patient-Reported Apnea Questionnaire (PRAQ) increase patient-centredness in the daily practice of sleep centres? a mixed-methods study. BMJ Open 2019; 9(6):e025963.

61. van Straten A, van der Zweerde T, Kleiboer A, et al. Cognitive and behavioral therapies in the treatment of insomnia: a meta-analysis. Sleep Med Rev 2018; 38:3–16.

62. Bastien CH, Vallieres A, Morin CM. Validation of the Insomnia Severity Index as an outcome measure for insomnia research. Sleep Med 2001;2(4):297–307.

63. Morin CM, Belleville G, Belanger L, et al. The Insomnia Severity Index: psychometric indicators to detect insomnia cases and evaluate treatment response. Sleep 2011;34(5):601–8.

64. Garcia-Borreguero D, Ferini-Strambi L, Kohnen R, et al. European guidelines on management of restless legs syndrome: report of a joint task force by the European Federation of Neurological Societies, the European Neurological Society and the European Sleep Research Society. Eur J Neurol 2012; 19(11):1385–96.

65. Abetz L, Vallow SM, Kirsch J, et al. Validation of the restless legs syndrome quality of life questionnaire. Value Health 2005;8(2):157–67.

66. Walters AS, LeBrocq C, Dhar A, et al. Validation of the international restless legs syndrome study group rating scale for restless legs syndrome. Sleep Med 2003;4(2):121–32.

67. Wolpert M. Uses and abuses of patient reported outcome measures (PROMs): potential iatrogenic impact of PROMs implementation and how it can be mitigated. Adm Policy Ment Health 2014;41(2): 141–5.

68. Janssen HCJP, Venekamp LN, Peeters GAM, et al. Management of insomnia in sleep disordered breathing. Eur Respir Rev 2019;28(153):190080.

69. Keenan BT, Kim J, Singh B, et al. Recognizable clinical subtypes of obstructive sleep apnea across international sleep centers: a cluster analysis. Sleep 2018;41(3):zsx214.

70. Smith AB, Hanbury A, Retzler J. Item banking and computer-adaptive testing in clinical trials: standing in sight of the PROMISed land. Contemp Clin Trials Commun 2019;13:005.

71. Buysse DJ, Yu L, Moul DE, et al. Development and validation of patient-reported outcome measures for sleep disturbance and sleep-related impairments. Sleep 2010;33(6):781–92.

Challenges and Opportunities for Applying Wearable Technology to Sleep

Selene Y. Tobin, MS[a], Paula G. Williams, PhD[b], Kelly G. Baron, PhD[c], Tanya M. Halliday, PhD[a], Christopher M. Depner, PhD[a],*

KEYWORDS

- Sleep loss • Sleep medicine • Biomarker • Circadian • Sleep disorder
- Circadian rhythm sleep-wake disorder • Consumer wearable • Actigraphy

KEY POINTS

- Wearable technology is in near ubiquitous use in modern society.
- Wearable technology for monitoring sleep is already being implemented in sleep medicine and research.
- The performance of most wearable devices designed to track sleep is not well-known, especially across different populations.
- This limited quantification of device performance in different populations is a primary factor limiting widespread use of wearable technologies in sleep medicine and research.

INTRODUCTION

The Sleep Research Society and American Academy of Sleep Medicine recommend adults regularly sleep at least 7 hours per night to promote optimal health.[1,2] Yet, approximately 1 in 3 adults in the United States report habitually sleeping less than this recommended 7 hours per night,[3–5] and approximately 50 to 70 million Americans suffer from chronic sleep disorders.[6] Epidemiologic findings from cross-sectional, case-control, prospective cohort, and meta-analysis studies show insufficient sleep is associated with risk of obesity, diabetes, cardiovascular disease, neurodegenerative disease, and psychological disorders.[7–13] Furthermore, findings from a Mendelian randomization study,[14] reflecting long-term exposure, suggest individuals with a genetic risk score associated with longer sleep duration have lower risk of congestive heart failure and hypertension. Finally, findings show experimentally imposed insufficient sleep in otherwise healthy adults leads to adverse changes in energy intake,[11,15–20] weight gain,[15,16,19] insulin sensitivity,[21–30] blood pressure,[31,32] inflammatory markers,[33–35] cognitive performance, and markers of neurodegenerative disorders, such as Alzheimer disease.[36,37] Multiple environmental, behavioral, or physiologic factors, including insufficient sleep schedules, social jetlag, circadian rhythm sleep-wake disorders (CRSWDs), shiftwork and shiftwork disorder, insomnia, sleep-disordered breathing, narcolepsy, and periodic limb movement disorder can contribute to habitual insufficient sleep. Given the high prevalence and range of causes of insufficient sleep, a priority is to develop sleep biomarkers with the goal of improving diagnosis, treatment, and prevention of sleep disruption.[38–40]

[a] Department of Health and Kinesiology, University of Utah, 250 S 1850 E, RM245, Salt Lake City, UT 84112, USA; [b] Department of Psychology, University of Utah, 380 S 1530 E Beh S 502, Salt Lake City, UT 84112, USA; [c] Division of Public Health, Department of Family and Preventative Medicine, University of Utah, 375 Chipeta Way Ste. A, Salt Lake City, UT 84108, USA
* Corresponding author. University of Utah, 250 S 1850 E; HPER North, RM 245, Salt Lake City, UT 84112, USA.
E-mail address: christopher.depner@utah.edu

Sleep Med Clin 16 (2021) 607–618
https://doi.org/10.1016/j.jsmc.2021.07.002
1556-407X/21/© 2021 Elsevier Inc. All rights reserved.

To optimize implementation, sleep biomarkers need to provide ecologically relevant (ie, free-living) data on multiple dimensions of sleep health that extend beyond sleep duration, such as regularity, satisfaction, alertness, timing, and efficiency.[41] The rapidly expanding wearable device technology represents on promising pipeline for developing sleep biomarkers. Wearable devices have a history in sleep research dating back to the 1970s when Foster and colleagues[42] showed a wrist-worn movement tracking device had potential for analyzing sleep and wakefulness. Following these initial findings Kripke and colleagues[43] published similar data in 1978 and referred to the methodology as "actigraphy." These studies paved the way for modern wrist actigraphy, which is commonly used and accepted for assessing free-living sleep and wakefulness in clinical and research settings.

MODERN WRIST ACTIGRAPHY AND CONSUMER WEARABLE DEVICES

Modern wrist actigraphy quantifies sleep by measuring body movements using triaxial accelerometry.[44–46] Many state-of-the-art actigraphs also measure light intensity. Despite technological enhancements in data collection and battery life, there are several barriers to widespread use and implementation of wrist actigraphy, including proprietary algorithms, relatively high cost, and the expertise required to analyze and interpret the data. Alternatively, consumer wearable devices are cheaper and easier to use, and most include additional physiologic and environmental measures, such as heart rate, electroencephalography (EEG), blood oxygen levels, geographic location, skin temperature, and noise (environmental and snoring). Furthermore, consumer wearable devices are nearly ubiquitous in modern society with approximately 125 million devices shipped in quarter 3 of 2020, representing approximately 35.1% growth over quarter 3 of 2019.[47] The wearable devices shipped in 2020 alone produced billions of nights of "sleep-tracking" data. Consumer wearable devices therefore represent a viable approach to overcome some limitations of wrist actigraphy. Yet, most consumer wearable devices still use proprietary algorithms and do not have Food and Drug Administration (FDA) clearance as medical devices, and therefore do not overcome all limitations of wrist actigraphy.

An international working group with experts in medical devices, sleep technology, sleep and circadian physiology, translational research, and sleep medicine met in 2018 to identify barriers for applying wearables to sleep and circadian science.[38] This working group identified the scarcity of independent validation studies designed to quantify performance of consumer wearable devices against accepted gold standards as the primary barrier for applying consumer wearables to sleep and circadian science.[38] The current gold standard for quantifying sleep is polysomnography (PSG), consisting of EEG, electromyography, electrooculography, electrocardiography (ECG), pulse oximetry, thoracic and abdominal effort belts, nasal air-flow sensors, and generally includes video and audio recordings to monitor body position, movements, and snoring.[48] Traditional PSG is conducted over a single night in clinical settings and is usually conducted for 1 to 5 nights in laboratory-controlled research settings. Thus, PSG is not designed or amenable to longitudinal sleep tracking over longer timeframes, especially for considering night-to-night variability. Directly translating PSG into wearable technology is challenging because of the extensive physiologic monitoring and complexity of interpreting PSG data. However, aspects of PSG, including blood oxygen saturation, EEG electrodes, heart rate, and snore microphones, are already incorporated into some consumer wearable devices.[38,49–53] An advantage of such wearable devices is the potential to track sleep longitudinally over months to years in ecologically relevant environments in thousands of individuals. On the other hand, many potential concerns still exist. For example, there are concerns for using microphones in wearable devices to detect snoring for assessment of obstructive sleep apnea, as it is possible for bed partners or ambient noise to impact the data. Although consumer wearable devices have potential to advance the field, each device and algorithm must undergo robust validation to quantify the performance of the device against relevant gold standards before clinical and research implementation (**Fig. 1**).

WEARABLE VALIDATION STUDIES
Performance of Wearable Devices to Assess Sleep Duration and Stages

See reviews by Baron and colleagues[49] and de Zambotti and colleagues[50] for extensive summaries of sleep wearable validation studies. Since the publication of these reviews, Chinoy and colleagues[51] published findings comparing the performance of 7 consumer sleep-tracking devices against PSG. Consistent with prior literature, Chinoy and colleagues[51] show consumer wearable devices tend to overestimate PSG total sleep time and underestimate PSG wakefulness after sleep onset. Although fewer data incorporate

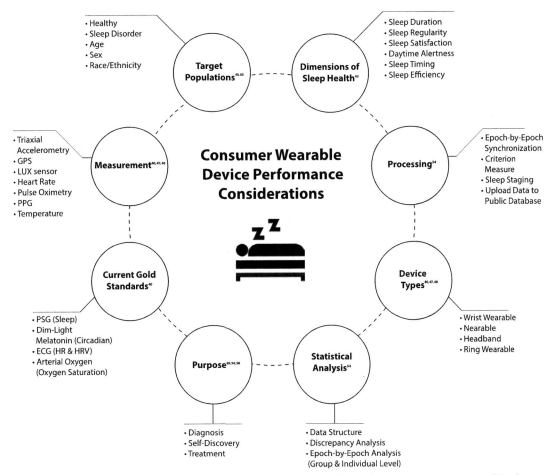

Fig. 1. Eight key considerations and associated variables of interest for performance assessments and implementation of sleep wearable devices. HR, heart rate.

epoch-by-epoch analyses, findings generally show wearable devices have high performance to classify PSG-defined sleep epochs (sensitivity), but low performance to classify PSG-defined wake epochs (specificity).[51] As such, wearable device performance generally decreases with worse sleep disruption and fragmentation, as observed in sleep disorders,[51] and it is therefore critical to conduct epoch-by-epoch analyses in validation studies to fully quantify device performance. For example, without conducting epoch-by-epoch analyses, it is impossible to understand the accuracy of a given device to identify the number and duration of awakenings across the night. Because these are essential metrics to understand for clinical diagnosis of sleep disorders, and these metrics are known to change across different populations, epoch-by-epoch analyses must be conducted before clinical implementation. Although not the gold standard, comparison against wrist actigraphy shows the performance

of most, but not all, consumer wearable devices to detect sleep versus wakefulness is similar to or better than wrist actigraphy.[51] Thus, in some instances, consumer wearable devices represent a viable option for tracking sleep and wakefulness in clinical or research settings, pending the population and intended use of the data (see **Fig. 1**).

A major limitation of most consumer wearable devices is their low performance to classify PSG-defined sleep stages. Most wearable devices with algorithms designed to classify sleep stages report estimates of light sleep, deep sleep, and rapid eye movement (REM) sleep. Light sleep presumably corresponds to stages N1 and N2 sleep and deep sleep corresponds to stage N3 sleep.[48] Most devices tend to overestimate light sleep (stages N1 and N2) and deep sleep (stage N3), underestimate REM sleep, and show high individual night variability.[51] These recent findings showing the limitations of consumer wearables to classify sleep stages, and the high variability between devices, support the 2018 international working group consensus that implementation of consumer wearables for sleep medicine and research is premature.[38] Some newer headband-type devices that incorporate EEG electrodes show promise for better sleep staging performance. The Dreem Headband is one such device that uses EEG, heart rate, movement (accelerometry), and a microphone (snoring) to estimate sleep staging and is a registered FDA class II medical device. Initial findings suggest the Dreem Headband has superior performance to most typical wrist-worn consumer wearable devices for classifying sleep stages.[52] However, such headband devices usually cost more than common wrist-worn consumer wearable devices, and thus the end-user must consider the strengths and limitations of each device.

Limitations and Needs of Current Wearables for Assessing Sleep Duration and Stages

Given the identified limitations with current wearable devices, a single device could have varying performance across different populations, such as adolescents, adults, or individuals with sleep disorders. Although performance assessments of any specific wearable device against PSG in mixed populations is limited, the performance of the Fitbit Flex is lower in individuals with insomnia versus healthy individuals,[54] and the performance of Fitbit Ultra changes across developmental age groups and with severity of sleep-disordered breathing in children and adolescents.[55] Specifically, the ability to detect wakefulness after sleep onset was lower in adolescents versus preschool and school-aged children, and differences between PSG and the Fitbit Ultra device were greater for children and adolescents with more severe sleep-disordered breathing.[55] These observations are further supported by findings showing sleep fragmentation decreases wearable device performance.[51] These findings highlight the need for comprehensive validation studies to define device performance in the specific population and environment of interest, such as older age, sleep disorders, or specific racial and ethnic backgrounds (see **Fig. 1**).

Despite published validation studies, on the whole, the rate of advancing technology in the consumer wearable industry greatly outpaces the capacity of clinicians and researchers to conduct robust validation studies. Furthermore, most wearable devices are classified as "wellness" products and are therefore not regulated by the FDA in the United States and cannot be used for clinical diagnosis or treatments. It is

therefore critical for researchers and clinicians to consider the use and implementation of wearable devices on a case-by-case basis to ensure the implemented device meets their required performance needs based on the population and outcome of interest. If validation and performance assessments are not published for a specific device or algorithm, it is best practice to conduct the necessary performance assessments before device implementation. Guidelines for conducting, reporting, and interpreting device performance studies are published.[38,56,57] Briefly, for designing and interpreting studies, these guidelines highlight the importance of comparing devices against established gold standards, defining and understanding the impact of different device settings (eg, normal vs sensitive), and defining the study sample. For analyzing and reporting data from performance studies, these guidelines highlight the importance of epoch-by-epoch analyses, use of consistent analyses across studies, publishing code for all analyses, making data freely available, and reporting the algorithm version and time frame of data collection because these parameters are continuously updated. Using these guidelines will facilitate systematic comparisons of device performance between studies and populations. In their recent publication, Menghini and colleagues[56,57] make the distinction between device "validation" versus device "performance" and recommend the field replaces the term "validity" with "performance" in this context. Notably, there are no consensus definitions for performance thresholds for any given device to be "validated" and such thresholds likely vary based on the population and outcome of interest. Such an approach to adopt the term "performance" allows the end-user, or regulatory bodies in the case of sleep medicine, to a priori establish performance thresholds.

Best practices and recommendations for clinical[58] and research[38] implementation of wearable devices have been published. Among these guidelines there is consensus to make data and algorithms from studies of sleep-tracking wearable devices freely available. A critical resource to accomplish this need is the development of a centralized repository for data management and access to code for sleep scoring algorithms. Developing and implementing such a resource has a high chance of leading to improved device performance and could allow the end-user to analyze data using the best-known algorithm for their population of interest. Such an approach also facilitates hypothesis generation and re-analysis of previous data with updated and better-performing algorithms as they are developed. Similar policies and resources for making data freely available have a history of advancing other fields, such as genomics, transcriptomics, proteomics, and metabolomics.[59,60]

Limitations and Needs of Current Wearables for Assessing Physiologic Endpoints Linked to Sleep

Physiologic measures beyond sleep and wakefulness also require validation. Recently, wearable devices have expanded their range of measures to include optical heart rate and heart rate variability (HRV) using photoplethysmography (PPG). These applications provide unique opportunities to access continuous and longitudinal heart rate and HRV data. Generally, heart rate and HRV data obtained from consumer wearables demonstrate good reliability and reproducibility when compared with ECG or previously validated chest-worn heart rate monitors.[61–64] However, suspected errors and shortcomings in these technologies potentially limit their reliability and have raised concern for exacerbating racial disparities and bias in health research and public policy.[65] Specifically, findings show skin tone can contribute to inaccurate PPG heart rate measurements, and particularly, reported errors occur more frequently when PPG is applied to individuals with dark versus light skin.[66,67] It is therefore critically important to quantify PPG performance across all skin tones and make necessary changes to ensure equitable implementation across racial and ethnic backgrounds. Other sources of potential error in capturing heart rate and HRV include motion artifact, which may be affected by displacement of the PPG sensor, blood flow dynamics, skin deformation, ambient temperature, wrist circumference, and biological sex.[63,68,69]

Another utility of PPG is assessing blood oxygen saturation. This is important for detecting sleep-disordered breathing, including obstructive sleep apnea.[70] Using PPG, several wearable devices provide insight into the user's blood oxygen saturation during sleep. Although such technology has potential benefit in detecting undiagnosed sleep-disordered breathing, due to the limitations explained previously, these measurements may not have the necessary performance or consistency across populations for research and/or clinical needs. Currently, there is a lack of studies and data assessing the performance of wearable devices versus clinical pulse oximetry to measure blood oxygen saturation and this is an urgently needed area of future research to properly inform the field on device performance.[65] Similar data

are also needed to determine the impact of anatomic location of the PPG on the human as it pertains to sleep-related outcomes, as data suggest performance can differ by body location (eg, finger vs wrist).[71] Another consideration for the sleep field is the use of transmission versus reflectance-based oximetry sensors.[72] Transmission-based sensors have 2 sides, are more common in clinical settings, and are limited to locations such as fingers, earlobes, and the nasal septum. Reflective-based sensors have only 1 side and thus can be placed in a range of body locations, including the wrist, and are therefore more common in free-living wearable devices. It is important to consider the potential differences in these sensor types as it relates to sleep physiology. To our knowledge, there are no systematic investigations of how these different sensor types may perform for the purpose of sleep wearables. Furthermore, recent findings suggest similar bias due to skin color may exist in pulse oximetry, which is commonly used for clinical diagnosis of sleep-disordered breathing.[73] These findings show there is an urgent need to perform robust assessments of PPG and pulse oximetry technologies in consumer and medical-grade wearable devices across different populations including diverse racial and ethnic backgrounds. Such information could inform technological advances to help combat health disparities.

USING WEARABLES TO ADDRESS SLEEP RESEARCH NEEDS

Sleep is multidimensional, including measures of total sleep time, regularity, alertness, timing, and efficiency.[41] Furthermore, data indicate that sleep is regulated by interactions between sleep homeostatic (process S) and circadian (process C) systems as posited by the 2-process model of sleep regulation.[74,75] Although the sleep and circadian fields have made extraordinary progress in understanding basic sleep and circadian physiology, there is a need to better understand the interactions between sleep and circadian physiology in ecologically relevant environments over timeframes of weeks to years. Despite the noted limitations, the rapidly progressing technology underlying consumer wearables represents an unprecedented opportunity to leverage this technology and advance the field. In the following, we highlight some key topics consumer wearable devices are well suited to help address.

Longitudinal Sleep Tracking

Because consumer wearables are in near ubiquitous use in modern society and are relatively inexpensive, this presents an opportunity to objectively quantify sleep physiology in thousands of individuals over weeks to years. Such data have the potential improve our understanding of how different sleep trajectories (eg, insufficient sleep during the workweek followed by weekend "recovery" sleep, or changes in sleep duration during the summer vs the academic year in adolescents) track with health outcomes, including cognitive performance, psychological disorders, and risk of cardiometabolic and neurodegenerative disorders. Furthermore, such data could inform our understanding of individual differences in physiologic and behavioral responses to sleep and circadian disruption, including long-term physiologic responses to exposures like working night shiftwork for multiple years. Such data could inform targeted sleep and circadian interventions designed to mitigate risk of chronic disease linked to poor sleep health.

Understanding Phenotypes of Habitual Short Sleepers

Most data linking short sleep duration with adverse health outcomes is derived from relatively small-sample, short-duration laboratory-controlled trials or large-scale epidemiologic studies. Data from laboratory protocols that experimentally restrict sleep in healthy adults, who normally sleep 7 hours or more per night, do not translate to individuals with habitual sleep durations of less than the recommended 7 hours per night. Alternatively, many epidemiologic studies rely on self-report questionnaires and lack objective sleep analyses, limiting interpretation of their findings. Prior data show approximately 1 in 3 individuals with habitual short sleep duration do not perceive or report daytime dysfunction related to their short sleep duration.[76] These data suggest there are at least 2 phenotypes of individuals with habitual short sleep duration, individuals with or without perceived daytime dysfunction. It is unknown if a lack of perceived daytime dysfunction among objectively verified habitual short sleepers confers protection against adverse health outcomes, such as cardiovascular disease. Large-scale representative samples collected over months to years are needed to characterize phenotypes in habitual short sleepers. Wearable devices offer the opportunity to advance research designed to identify factors contributing to variation in sleep-related daytime dysfunction in real-world environments. Advancements in wearable technology, including incorporation of additional physiologic monitoring capabilities, such as global positioning system (GPS), PPG, and EEG, when

validated, could provide real-world, ecologically relevant data to better understand mechanisms underlying habitual short-sleeper phenotypes and related health outcomes.

Linking Changes in Multiple Dimensions of Sleep Physiology with Changes in Health Outcomes

Because sleep is not a static process and is under homeostatic regulation, there is a need to better understand how different dimensions of sleep relate to adverse health outcomes over months to years. For example, sleep fragmentation,[77] slow-wave sleep suppression,[78] and disrupted circadian timing of wakefulness during insufficient sleep[24] can each contribute to impaired insulin sensitivity. Yet, it is not well understood how disruption of any one specific sleep dimension over months to years may differentially impact health outcomes compared with disruption of a different sleep dimension over the same timeframe (eg, effects of fragmented sleep vs insufficient sleep opportunities on insulin sensitivity over months to years). One approach to target this question is to integrate data derived from wearable devices with omics-based biomarker data to understand how different biochemical pathways are impacted by different sleep dimensions. Such omics-based data relevant to insufficient sleep in the laboratory setting are published.[79,80] Integrating wearable-based with omics-based data represent a logical next step to conduct studies in ecologically relevant settings over longer durations. This approach could inform new interventions that target specific dimensions of sleep health based on individual risk profiles.

Analyzing Circadian Timing Under Free-living Conditions

Chang and colleagues[81] recently published findings using standard wrist actigraphy data to predict circadian phase measured by dim-light melatonin onset. In addition, findings also suggest changes in skin temperature can be measured and used to estimate changes in core body temperature and thus could potentially help inform assessments of circadian timing.[82] If validated in independent cohorts, such as free-living shiftworkers and individuals with sleep disorders, it is possible that the current technology may be adequate for assessing circadian phase. However, if such independent performance assessments show that the current technology is not adequate, other metrics and innovative technological advances may be required (eg, real-time blood sampling[83,84]) to measure circadian-regulated metabolites or gene expression that could improve accuracy of wearable technologies. Despite these promising findings and the importance of circadian timing to sleep regulation and overall health, few wearable devices are designed to assess circadian timing.[38] Thus, there is a need and opportunity to develop consumer wearable devices and related technology designed to measure circadian timing in ecologically relevant environments over months to years.

Tracking Heart Rate Variability as a Marker of Stress Load

HRV, the fluctuation in length of heart-beat intervals, is an established measure of the autonomic nervous system.[85] HRV has therefore emerged as a noninvasive biomarker of overall stress load.[86] Bidirectional relationships exist between perceived stress and self-reported or actigraphy measured sleep.[87,88] For instance, findings show self-reported stress negatively impacts sleep quantity and quality, and poor sleep can increase next-day perceived stress.[89] Furthermore, a single HRV measurement collected in the resting, wakeful state was associated with sleep-diary–reported sleep efficiency in one trial of healthy, college-aged men.[90] These findings highlight the potential to use HRV measurement in wearable devices to objectively measure stress levels in free-living settings and better understand potential mechanisms linking stress and the multiple dimensions of sleep. In addition, wearable devices can be used in interventions to determine the causal impact of stress reduction on sleep outcomes as well as sleep extension on stress reduction. Finally, wearable devices can be used for the duration of clinical trials, allowing better evaluation of the time course of responses compared with standard laboratory-based assessments conducted at baseline and postintervention only.

Using Global Positioning System to Determine Participant Location Within and Across Time Zones

The timing of sunrise and sunset (ie, duration of sunlight) are powerful cues (zeitgebers) for the circadian clock.[91,92] Misalignment between the light-dark cycle (or behavioral cycle) and the master circadian clock lead to adverse health outcomes.[11] The social construction of time zones results in heterogeneity of the actual clock hour of sunrise and sunset within a given time zone, with sunrise and sunset occurring more than 1 hour earlier on the eastern edge compared with the western edge of many time zones.[93] The later evening sunlight that is present farther west in a time zone is associated with reduced sleep duration and adverse health outcomes, such as obesity, diabetes, myocardial infarction, and cancer.[94,95] Related, individuals that live near the borders of time zones, or who frequently travel across time zones (eg, live in Indiana, but work in Illinois) may be uniquely influenced by daily living across 2 "social clocks." It is currently unknown how habitual, daily time zone shifts impact the links between sleep and other health-related behaviors, and therefore health outcomes. The GPS capabilities available in wearable devices could be used to fill these gaps in knowledge and support the creation of evidence-based best practices in behavioral sleep medicine.

CLINICAL CARE POINTS
Objective Assessment of Insomnia

Tracking sleep with traditional handwritten sleep logs is a foundational tool of behavioral sleep medicine and use of research-grade actigraphy is an important diagnostic tool for populations with limited ability to self-report their sleep, such as people with dementia and children.[46] According to the American Academy of Sleep Medicine practice parameters, use of research-grade actigraphy is an option for patients with insomnia but not a standard recommendation in treatment. Consumer wearable devices have the potential to replace or at least complement the use of sleep logs and actigraphy; however, when being used to inform clinical diagnoses, it is imperative that the wearable device provides accurate sleep-tracking data. As noted, the rate of validation and performance assessment studies cannot keep up with the pace of new technology in consumer wearable devices and therefore the performance of many consumer wearable devices in specific patient populations is not well characterized. This may limit the clinical effectiveness of using such devices. On the other hand, given the widespread use of consumer wearable devices, there is potential opportunity for these devices to detect possible undiagnosed sleep disorders. Under such circumstances, if this information is transferred to a primary care provider, then the potential sleep disorder could be identified and followed-up on accordingly.

Enhanced Understanding of Circadian Rhythm Sleep-Wake Disorders

CRSWDs are a class of sleep disorders in which sleep and wakefulness occur at irregular or abnormal times and typically result in insomnia, excessive daytime sleepiness, or both. Estimates show approximately 800,000 to 3,000,000 people suffer from CRSWDs in the United States.[96] CRSWDs are believed to arise from misalignment of the circadian and behavioral (environmental) cycles, alterations in the circadian system itself, or dysfunction of the entrainment mechanisms of the circadian system.[70] A 2019 working group identified the poor understanding about the cause, prevalence, time course, and comorbidities of CRSWDs as a major knowledge gap limiting effective treatment.[96] For example, prior findings show some patients with CRSWD have apparently normal timing of their circadian clock, yet have abnormal or irregular sleep timing,[97] potentially contributing to poor treatment efficacy. Such data highlight our incomplete understanding of the pathophysiological basis of CRSWD. One of the biggest challenges with diagnosing and treating CRSWD is that the current gold standard for assessing the circadian clock, dim-light melatonin assessment, is burdensome, expensive, time-consuming, and does not have established clinically normal values.[96] Ultimately, a lack of biomarkers for measuring circadian timing under free-living conditions is a primary factor contributing to this knowledge gap. Given their widespread use, wearable devices are well positioned to help address this knowledge gap. For example, some data show measuring skin temperature can be used to estimate changes in core body temperature and therefore circadian timing.[82] In addition, omics-based biomarkers designed to measure the master circadian clock are being developed,[84,98] and integrating these omics-based biomarkers with wearable devices that can accurately track behaviors (sleep-wake timing) over weeks to months could further help address this knowledge gap. However, these omics-based biomarkers and wearable devices require further validation studies to assess their performance in broader populations before such implementation is possible. Although much work remains for developing wearable devices that track circadian timing, wearables in general are an attractive option for addressing the key knowledge gaps in CRSWD. Continued effort in this area is warranted, as an improved understanding of CRSWDs has high potential to lead to improved treatment strategies.

Just-In-Time Feedback to Clinicians

Another potential advantage of use of wearable technology is the ability for patients to share their data and adjust the timing of treatment. Two-way communication between patients and clinicians is not feasible with existing actigraphy devices. Traditional actigraphy requires the patient to pick up the device and return to the clinic for download, rather than real-time review. Some laboratories are developing just-in-time adaptive interventions that use self-report and wearable data, combined with 2-way messaging to deliver interventions.[99] This type of intervention may be particularly useful for patients with CRSWD using melatonin or bright-light therapies because the treatment response occurs rapidly and may require clinician feedback to adjust the timing. However, the return visit to the clinic may not occur for weeks, or months. In addition, the use of oximetry data (although not clinically validated yet) could provide information regarding the efficacy of treatments with continuous positive airway pressure devices. Relevant to insomnia, some behavioral insomnia research programs have incorporated consumer wearable devices and demonstrate feasibility of using devices in these programs.[99,100] However, it is not known if using a wearable device enhances treatment outcomes in these settings.[101]

Enhancing Behavior Change, Particularly for Short Sleepers

Prior research regarding the acceptability of devices suggests they are a favored treatment, particularly among short sleepers who are interested in extending their sleep.[102] For example, findings show simple techniques such as goal setting and brief telephone coaching can encourage short sleepers to extend their sleep.[103,104] Use of sleep-tracking technology is a key feature of the treatment and regarded by patients as the most enjoyable aspect of the intervention.

SUMMARY

The rapidly progressing wearable device industry is presenting clinicians and researchers with unprecedented opportunity to translate basic sleep research findings into clinical practice. Equally important, the public has already embraced the "self-quantification" movement and the use of wearable devices in modern society is nearly ubiquitous. One of the primary remaining barriers for sleep clinicians and researchers to leverage commercial wearable devices is the general lack of validation and performance assessments of such devices. Because best practices for validation and performance assessment studies are already published,[50,56] we highlighted the key considerations for performance assessment and implementation of wearable devices for sleep medicine and research (see **Fig. 1**). We also identified some key pitfalls in device performance, notably potential racial and ethnic bias in PPG and pulse oximetry, and a general lack of performance assessments in populations with sleep disorders. Although some devices do track circadian timing, there is a broad lack of devices that can measure circadian timing with the needed performance for clinical and research purposes. Despite the limitations, consumer wearable devices are already being implemented in sleep medicine and research and we anticipate this trend will continue upward. As a field, the onus is on sleep clinicians and researchers to maintain the rigor and performance of current gold standards, such as PSG, that provided the knowledge base for the rapid development of the wearable device industry. Given the range of adverse health consequences linked with sleep and circadian disruption and the rapidly evolving wearable device technology, researchers and clinicians will likely always need to make case-by-case decisions on the best device for their outcome of interest. When the noted limitations are overcome, the sleep field is well poised to make great advances in knowledge and clinical care by leveraging the power of wearables.

DISCLOSURE

P.G. Williams was supported by resources from the University of Utah Neuroscience Initiative. K.G. Baron reports receiving research support from the National Institutes of Health (NIH) (R01NR018891); T.M. Halliday reports receiving support from the NIH (KL2TR002539); C.M. Depner reports receiving support from the NIH (K01HL145099), the Colorado Clinical and Translational Sciences Institute, and the University of Utah Vice President for Research Seed Grant Program, and Consulting fees from Elsevier Inc that are unrelated to this work.

REFERENCES

1. Watson NF, Badr MS, Belenky G, et al. Recommended amount of sleep for a healthy adult: a joint consensus statement of the American Academy of Sleep Medicine and Sleep Research Society. Sleep 2015;38(6):843–4.
2. Watson NF, Badr MS, Belenky G, et al. Recommended amount of sleep for a healthy adult: a joint consensus statement of the American Academy of Sleep Medicine and Sleep Research Society. J Clin Sleep Med 2015;11(6):591–2.
3. Ford ES, Cunningham TJ, Croft JB. Trends in self-reported sleep duration among US adults from 1985 to 2012. Sleep 2015;38(5):829–32.
4. Centers for Disease Control and Prevention. Effect of short sleep duration on daily activities–United States, 2005-2008. Morb Mortal Wkly Rep 2011; 60(8):239–42.
5. Centers for Disease Control and Prevention. Short sleep duration among US adults 2014. Available at: https://www.cdc.gov/sleep/data_statistics.html. Accessed September 24, 2018.
6. Colten HR, editor. Sleep disorders and sleep deprivation: an unmet public health problem. Washington, DC: National Academies Press; 2006.
7. Cappuccio FP, Cooper D, D'Elia L, et al. Sleep duration predicts cardiovascular outcomes: a systematic review and meta-analysis of prospective studies. Eur Heart J 2011;32(12):1484–92.
8. Cappuccio FP, D'Elia L, Strazzullo P, et al. Quantity and quality of sleep and incidence of type 2 diabetes: a systematic review and meta-analysis. Diabetes Care 2010;33(2):414–20.
9. Cappuccio FP, Taggart FM, Kandala NB, et al. Meta-analysis of short sleep duration and obesity in children and adults. Sleep 2008;31(5):619–26.
10. Holliday EG, Magee CA, Kritharides L, et al. Short sleep duration is associated with risk of future diabetes but not cardiovascular disease: a prospective study and meta-analysis. PLoS One 2013; 8(11):e82305.
11. Depner CM, Stothard ER, Wright KP Jr. Metabolic consequences of sleep and circadian disorders. Curr Diab Rep 2014;14(7):507.
12. St-Onge MP, Grandner MA, Brown D, et al. Sleep duration and quality: impact on lifestyle behaviors and cardiometabolic health: a scientific statement from the American Heart Association. Circulation 2016;134(18):e367–86.
13. Lucey BP. It's complicated: the relationship between sleep and Alzheimer's disease in humans. Neurobiol Dis 2020;144:105031.
14. Dashti HS, Redline S, Saxena R. Polygenic risk score identifies associations between sleep duration and diseases determined from an electronic medical record biobank. Sleep 2018;42(3):zsy247.
15. Markwald RR, Melanson EL, Smith MR, et al. Impact of insufficient sleep on total daily energy expenditure, food intake, and weight gain. Proc Natl Acad Sci U S A 2013;110(14):5695–700.
16. Bosy-Westphal A, Hinrichs S, Jauch-Chara K, et al. Influence of partial sleep deprivation on energy balance and insulin sensitivity in healthy women. Obes Facts 2008;1(5):266–73.
17. Brondel L, Romer MA, Nougues PM, et al. Acute partial sleep deprivation increases food intake in healthy men. Am J Clin Nut 2010;91(6):1550–9.
18. Nedeltcheva AV, Kilkus JM, Imperial J, et al. Sleep curtailment is accompanied by increased intake of calories from snacks. Am J Clin Nut 2009;89(1): 126–33.
19. Spaeth AM, Dinges DF, Goel N. Effects of experimental sleep restriction on weight gain, caloric

intake, and meal timing in healthy adults. Sleep 2013;36(7):981–90.

20. St-Onge MP, Roberts AL, Chen J, et al. Short sleep duration increases energy intakes but does not change energy expenditure in normal-weight individuals. Am J Clin Nut 2011;94(2):410–6.

21. Donga E, van Dijk M, van Dijk JG, et al. A single night of partial sleep deprivation induces insulin resistance in multiple metabolic pathways in healthy subjects. J Clin Endocrinol Metab 2010;95(6):2963–8.

22. Rao MN, Neylan TC, Grunfeld C, et al. Subchronic sleep restriction causes tissue-specific insulin resistance. J Clin Endocrinol Metab 2015;100(4):1664–71.

23. Broussard JL, Chapotot F, Abraham V, et al. Sleep restriction increases free fatty acids in healthy men. Diabetologia 2015;58(4):791–8.

24. Eckel RH, Depner CM, Perreault L, et al. Morning circadian misalignment during short sleep duration impacts insulin sensitivity. Curr Bio 2015;25(22):3004–10.

25. Broussard JL, Ehrmann DA, Van Cauter E, et al. Impaired insulin signaling in human adipocytes after experimental sleep restriction: a randomized, crossover study. Ann Intern Med 2012;157(8):549–57.

26. Spiegel K, Leproult R, Van Cauter E. Impact of sleep debt on metabolic and endocrine function. Lancet 1999;354(9188):1435–9.

27. Buxton OM, Pavlova M, Reid EW, et al. Sleep restriction for 1 week reduces insulin sensitivity in healthy men. Diabetes 2010;59(9):2126–33.

28. Leproult R, Holmback U, Van Cauter E. Circadian misalignment augments markers of insulin resistance and inflammation, independently of sleep loss. Diabetes 2014;63(6):1860–9.

29. Nedeltcheva AV, Kessler L, Imperial J, et al. Exposure to recurrent sleep restriction in the setting of high caloric intake and physical inactivity results in increased insulin resistance and reduced glucose tolerance. J Clin Endocrinol Metab 2009;94(9):3242–50.

30. Depner CM, Melanson EL, Eckel RH, et al. Ad libitum weekend recovery sleep fails to prevent metabolic dysregulation during a repeating pattern of insufficient sleep and weekend recovery sleep. Curr Bio 2019;29(6):957–67.e4.

31. Robillard R, Lanfranchi PA, Prince F, et al. Sleep deprivation increases blood pressure in healthy normotensive elderly and attenuates the blood pressure response to orthostatic challenge. Sleep 2011;34(3):335–9.

32. Yang H, Haack M, Gautam S, et al. Repetitive exposure to shortened sleep leads to blunted sleep-associated blood pressure dipping. J Hypertens 2017;35(6):1187–94.

33. Frey DJ, Fleshner M, Wright KP Jr. The effects of 40 hours of total sleep deprivation on inflammatory markers in healthy young adults. Brain Behav Immun 2007;21(8):1050–7.

34. Meier-Ewert HK, Ridker PM, Rifai N, et al. Effect of sleep loss on C-reactive protein, an inflammatory marker of cardiovascular risk. J Am Coll Cardiol 2004;43(4):678–83.

35. van Leeuwen WM, Lehto M, Karisola P, et al. Sleep restriction increases the risk of developing cardiovascular diseases by augmenting proinflammatory responses through IL-17 and CRP. PLoS One 2009;4(2):e4589.

36. Barthelemy NR, Liu H, Lu W, et al. Sleep deprivation affects tau phosphorylation in human cerebrospinal fluid. Ann Neurol 2020;87(5):700–9.

37. Holth JK, Fritschi SK, Wang C, et al. The sleep-wake cycle regulates brain interstitial fluid tau in mice and CSF tau in humans. Science 2019;363(6429):880–4.

38. Depner CM, Cheng PC, Devine JK, et al. Wearable technologies for developing sleep and circadian biomarkers: a summary of workshop discussions. Sleep 2019;43(2):zsz254.

39. Mullington J, Pack AI, Ginsburg GS. In pursuit of sleep-circadian biomarkers. Sleep 2015;38(11):1665–6.

40. Mullington JM, Abbott SM, Carroll JE, et al. Developing biomarker arrays predicting sleep and circadian-coupled risks to health. Sleep 2016;39(4):727–36.

41. Buysse DJ. Sleep health: can we define it? Does it matter? Sleep 2014;37(1):9–17.

42. Foster FG, Kupfer D, Weiss G, et al. Mobility recording and cycle research in neuropsychiatry. J Interdiscip Cycle Res 1972;3(1):61–72.

43. Kripke DF, Mullaney DJ, Messin S, et al. Wrist actigraphic measures of sleep and rhythms. Electroencephalogr Clin Neurophysiol 1978;44(5):674–6.

44. Cole RJ, Kripke DF, Gruen W, et al. Automatic sleep/wake identification from wrist activity. Sleep 1992;15(5):461–9.

45. Ancoli-Israel S, Cole R, Alessi C, et al. The role of actigraphy in the study of sleep and circadian rhythms. Sleep 2003;26(3):342–92.

46. Morgenthaler T, Alessi C, Friedman L, et al. Practice parameters for the use of actigraphy in the assessment of sleep and sleep disorders: an update for 2007. Sleep 2007;30(4):519–29.

47. International Data Corporation. Shipments of wearable devices leap to 125 million units, up 35.1% in the third quarter, according to IDC 2020. Available at: https://www.idc.com/getdoc.jsp?containerId=prUS47067820#:~:text=FRAMINGHAM%2C%20Mass.%2C%20December%202,Worldwide%20Quarterly%20Wearable%20Device%20Tracker. Accessed March 10, 2021.

48. Berry RB, Albertario CL, Harding SM, et al. The AASM manual for the scoring of sleep and associated events: rules, terminology and technical specifications version 2.5. Darien, IL: American Academy of Sleep Medicine; 2018.

49. Baron KG, Duffecy J, Berendsen MA, et al. Feeling validated yet? A scoping review of the use of consumer-targeted wearable and mobile technology to measure and improve sleep. Sleep Med Rev 2018;40:151–9.

50. de Zambotti M, Cellini N, Goldstone A, et al. Wearable sleep technology in clinical and research settings. Med Sci Sports Exerc 2019;51(7):1538–57.

51. Chinoy ED, Cuellar JA, Huwa KE, et al. Performance of seven consumer sleep-tracking devices compared with polysomnography. Sleep 2020; 44(5):zsaa291.

52. Arnal PJ, Thorey V, Debellemaniere E, et al. The Dreem Headband compared to polysomnography for electroencephalographic signal acquisition and sleep staging. Sleep 2020;43(11):zsaa097.

53. Diep C, Garcia-Molina G, Jasko J, et al. Acoustic enhancement of slow wave sleep on consecutive nights improves alertness and attention in chronically short sleepers. Sleep Med 2021;81:69–79.

54. Kang SG, Kang JM, Ko KP, et al. Validity of a commercial wearable sleep tracker in adult insomnia disorder patients and good sleepers. J Psychosom Res 2017;97:38–44.

55. Meltzer LJ, Hiruma LS, Avis K, et al. Comparison of a commercial accelerometer with polysomnography and actigraphy in children and adolescents. Sleep 2015;38(8):1323–30.

56. Menghini L, Cellini N, Goldstone A, et al. A standardized framework for testing the performance of sleep-tracking technology: step-by-step guidelines and open-source code. Sleep 2021; 44(2):zsaa170.

57. Goldstein CA, Depner C. Miles to go before we sleep...a step toward transparent evaluation of consumer sleep tracking devices. Sleep 2021; 44(2):zsab020.

58. Khosla S, Deak MC, Gault D, et al. Consumer sleep technology: an American Academy of Sleep Medicine position statement. J Clin Sleep Med 2018; 14(5):877–80.

59. Piwowar HA, Becich MJ, Bilofsky H, et al. Intellectual Capital W. Towards a data sharing culture: recommendations for leadership from academic health centers. PLoS Med 2008;5(9):e183.

60. Chervitz SA, Deutsch EW, Field D, et al. Data standards for omics data: the basis of data sharing and reuse. Methods Mol Biol 2011;719:31–69.

61. Nelson BW, Allen NB. Accuracy of consumer wearable heart rate measurement during an ecologically valid 24-hour period: intraindividual validation study. JMIR Mhealth Uhealth 2019;7(3):e10828.

62. Fuller D, Colwell E, Low J, et al. Reliability and validity of commercially available wearable devices for measuring steps, energy expenditure, and heart rate: systematic review. JMIR Mhealth Uhealth 2020;8(9):e18694.

63. Dobbs WC, Fedewa MV, MacDonald HV, et al. The accuracy of acquiring heart rate variability from portable devices: a systematic review and meta-analysis. Sports Med 2019;49(3):417–35.

64. Kinnunen H, Rantanen A, Kentta T, et al. Feasible assessment of recovery and cardiovascular health: accuracy of nocturnal HR and HRV assessed via ring PPG in comparison to medical grade ECG. Physiol Meas 2020;41(4):04NT01.

65. Colvonen PJ, DeYoung PN, Bosompra NA, et al. Limiting racial disparities and bias for wearable devices in health science research. Sleep 2020; 43(10):zsaa159.

66. Fallow BA, Tarumi T, Tanaka H. Influence of skin type and wavelength on light wave reflectance. J Clin Monit Comput 2013;27(3):313–7.

67. Shcherbina A, Mattsson CM, Waggott D, et al. Accuracy in wrist-worn, sensor-based measurements of heart rate and energy expenditure in a diverse cohort. J Pers Med 2017;7(2):3.

68. Castaneda D, Esparza A, Ghamari M, et al. A review on wearable photoplethysmography sensors and their potential future applications in health care. Int J Biosens Bioelectron 2018;4(4): 195–202.

69. Menghini L, Gianfranchi E, Cellini N, et al. Stressing the accuracy: wrist-worn wearable sensor validation over different conditions. Psychophysiology 2019;56(11):e13441.

70. International classification of sleep disorders. 3rd edition. Darien, IL: American Academy of Sleep Medicine; 2014.

71. Longmore SK, Lui GY, Naik G, et al. A comparison of reflective photoplethysmography for detection of heart rate, blood oxygen saturation, and respiration rate at various anatomical locations. Sensors 2019; 19(8):1874.

72. Berkenbosch JW, Tobias JD. Comparison of a new forehead reflectance pulse oximeter sensor with a conventional digit sensor in pediatric patients. Respir Care 2006;51(7):726–31.

73. Sjoding MW, Dickson RP, Iwashyna TJ, et al. Racial bias in pulse oximetry measurement. N Engl J Med 2020;383(25):2477–8.

74. Borbely AA. A two process model of sleep regulation. Hum Neurobiol 1982;1(3):195–204.

75. Borbely AA, Daan S, Wirz-Justice A, et al. The two-process model of sleep regulation: a reappraisal. J Sleep Res 2016;25(2):131–43.

76. Curtis BJ, Williams PG, Jones CR, et al. Sleep duration and resting fMRI functional connectivity: examination of short sleepers with and without

perceived daytime dysfunction. Brain Behav 2016; 6(12):e00576.

77. Stamatakis KA, Punjabi NM. Effects of sleep fragmentation on glucose metabolism in normal subjects. Chest 2010;137(1):95–101.

78. Tasali E, Leproult R, Ehrmann DA, et al. Slow-wave sleep and the risk of type 2 diabetes in humans. Proc Natl Acad Sci U S A 2008;105(3):1044–9.

79. Depner CM, Cogswell DT, Bisesi PJ, et al. Developing preliminary blood metabolomics-based biomarkers of insufficient sleep in humans. Sleep 2020;43(7):zsz321.

80. Laing EE, Moller-Levet CS, Dijk DJ, et al. Identifying and validating blood mRNA biomarkers for acute and chronic insufficient sleep in humans: a machine learning approach. Sleep 2019;42(1):zsy186.

81. Cheng P, Walch O, Huang Y, et al. Predicting circadian misalignment with wearable technology: validation of wrist-worn actigraphy and photometry in night shift workers. Sleep 2021;44(2):zsaa180.

82. McHill AW, Smith BJ, Wright KP Jr. Effects of caffeine on skin and core temperatures, alertness, and recovery sleep during circadian misalignment. J Biol Rhythms 2014;29(2):131–43.

83. Cogswell D, Bisesi P, Markwald RR, et al. Identification of a preliminary plasma metabolome-based biomarker for circadian phase in humans. J Biol Rhythms 2021;36(4):369–83.

84. Wittenbrink N, Ananthasubramaniam B, Munch M, et al. High-accuracy determination of internal circadian time from a single blood sample. J Clin Invest 2018;128(9):3826–39.

85. Heart rate variability. Standards of measurement, physiological interpretation, and clinical use. Task Force of the European Society of Cardiology and the North American Society of Pacing and Electrophysiology. Eur Heart J 1996;17(3):354–81.

86. Kim HG, Cheon EJ, Bai DS, et al. Stress and heart rate variability: a meta-analysis and review of the literature. Psychiatry Investig 2018;15(3):235–45.

87. Lee S, Crain TL, McHale SM, et al. Daily antecedents and consequences of nightly sleep. J Sleep Res 2017;26(4):498–509.

88. Vandekerckhove M, Cluydts R. The emotional brain and sleep: an intimate relationship. Sleep Med Rev 2010;14(4):219–26.

89. Yap Y, Slavish DC, Taylor DJ, et al. Bi-directional relations between stress and self-reported and actigraphy-assessed sleep: a daily intensive longitudinal study. Sleep 2020;43(3):zsz250.

90. Gouin JW K, Deschenes S, Dang-Vu T. Heart rate variability predicts sleep efficiency. Sleep Med 2013;14:e142.

91. Stothard ER, McHill AW, Depner CM, et al. Circadian entrainment to the natural light-dark cycle across seasons and the weekend. Curr Bio 2017; 27(4):508–13.

92. Wright KP Jr, McHill AW, Birks BR, et al. Entrainment of the human circadian clock to the natural light-dark cycle. Curr Bio 2013;23(16):1554–8.

93. Roenneberg T, Winnebeck EC, Klerman EB. Daylight saving time and artificial time zones - a battle between biological and social times. Front Physiol 2019;10:944.

94. Guintella OM F. Sunset time and the economic effects of social jetlag: evidence from US time zone borders. J Health Econ 2019;65:210–26.

95. Gu F, Xu S, Devesa SS, et al. Longitude position in a time zone and cancer risk in the United States. Cancer Epidemiol Biomarkers Prev 2017;26(8):1306–11.

96. Duffy JF, Abbott SM, Burgess HJ, et al. Workshop report. Circadian rhythm sleep-wake disorders: gaps and opportunities. Sleep 2021;44(5):zsaa281.

97. Rahman SA, Kayumov L, Tchmoutina EA, et al. Clinical efficacy of dim light melatonin onset testing in diagnosing delayed sleep phase syndrome. Sleep Med 2009;10(5):549–55.

98. Laing EE, Moller-Levet CS, Poh N, et al. Blood transcriptome based biomarkers for human circadian phase. eLife 2017;6:e20214.

99. Pulantara IW, Parmanto B, Germain A. Development of a just-in-time adaptive mHealth intervention for insomnia: usability study. JMIR Hum Factors 2018;5(2):e21.

100. Kang SG, Kang JM, Cho SJ, et al. Cognitive behavioral therapy using a mobile application synchronizable with wearable devices for insomnia treatment: a pilot study. J Clin Sleep Med 2017; 13(4):633–40.

101. Baron KGC LC, Duffecy J. How are consumer sleep technology data being used to deliver behavioral sleep medicine interventions? A systematic review. J Behav Sleep Med 2021;1–15.

102. Adkins EC, DeYonker O, Duffecy J, et al. Predictors of intervention interest among individuals with short sleep duration. J Clin Sleep Med 2019;15(8):1143–8.

103. Baron KG, Duffecy J, Richardson D, et al. Technology assisted behavior intervention to extend sleep among adults with short sleep duration and prehypertension/stage 1 hypertension: a randomized pilot feasibility study. J Clin Sleep Med 2019;15(11):1587–97.

104. Baron KG, Duffecy J, Reid K, et al. Technology-assisted behavioral intervention to extend sleep duration: development and design of the sleep bunny mobile app. JMIR Ment Health 2018;5(1):e3.

New Paths in Respiratory Sleep Medicine
Consumer Devices, e-Health, and Digital Health Measurements

Thomas Penzel, PhD[a,b,*], Sarah Dietz-Terjung, MSc[c], Holger Woehrle, MD[d],
Christoph Schöbel, MD, PhD[c]

KEYWORDS

- E-health • Out-of-center testing • Health apps • Longtime monitoring • Diagnostics
- Sleep-disordered breathing

KEY POINTS

- Severity assessment in sleep-disordered breathing needs more than the apnea-hypopnea index.
- Diagnostic tools use contact-free measurement of sleep and breathing at the home sleeping place.
- Wearables tracking sleep apnea activity may help in phenotyping sleep apnea as a diagnosis.
- Electronic health and digital health solutions provide support for conventional sleep medicine and promote the attention to care for good and healthy sleep.

INTRODUCTION

Sleep medicine is one of the most expanding fields in medicine of the past decades. It has its origins in sleep research and still is a new and highly interdisciplinary science. New developments are driven mainly by findings in physiology and pathophysiology as well as in diagnostics, therapy, and management of sleep-disordered breathing (SDB). From the beginning, sleep medicine has been characterized by quickly taking up new technical developments.

The field of respiratory sleep medicine is becoming increasingly important due to the rising prevalence of SDB.[1–3] The term SDB is used to describe breathing disorders during sleep. A distinction is made between pauses in breathing, apnea events, and reductions in respiratory flow with accompanying oxygen desaturations, and hypopnea events. The severity of SDB is determined by the apnea-hypopnea index (AHI)—the number of apnea and hypopnea events per hour of sleep: an AHI of 5/h to 15/h defines a mild graded SDB, whereas an AHI of 15/h to 30/h defines a moderate graded SDB; a severe graded SDB is diagnosed by an AHI of greater than 30/h.

The most common form of SDB is called obstructive sleep apnea (OSA): during sleep, the upper airways collapses, causing breathing disorders during sleep. Another form, central sleep apnea (CSA), is less common: here, the respiratory center in the brain stem briefly stops sending signals to the respiratory muscles during sleep.

SDBs lead to a reduced oxygen supply and causes physical stress due to short wake-up reactions or arousals, which are intended to prevent suffocation during sleep. In the short term, this leads to nonrestorative sleep with impaired physical and mental performance or even daytime

[a] Interdisciplinary Sleep Medicine Center, Charité – Universitätsmedizin Berlin, Freie Universität Berlin, Humboldt-Universität zu Berlin, Berlin Institute of Health, Berlin, Germany; [b] Department of Biology, Saratov State University, Astrakhanskaya Str. 12, Saratov 410012, Russia; [c] Universitätsmedizin Essen, Ruhrlandklinik, Westdeutsches Lungenzentrum am Universitätsklinikum Essen gGmbH, Tüschener Weg 40, 45239 Essen, Germany; [d] Lungenzentrum Ulm, Olgastr. 83, 89073 Ulm, Germany

* Corresponding author. Charite University Medicine, Sleep Medicine Center, Charitéplatz 1, Berlin 10117, Germany.

E-mail address: thomas.penzel@charite.de

Sleep Med Clin 16 (2021) 619–634
https://doi.org/10.1016/j.jsmc.2021.08.006

sleepiness. In the long term, untreated SDB increases the risk of cardiovascular disease or even dementia.

The problem is that sleep physicians currently are poor at assessing individual long-term risk in a patient with an elevated AHI. The level of the AHI, for example, only allows an inadequate individual risk assessment.

Typical symptoms of an untreated OSA include snoring, daytime sleepiness, and breathing cessations during sleep witnessed by bed partners)—leading to the term, OSA syndrome (OSAS). Not everyone with a diagnosed OSA based on an elevated AHI, however, shows typical symptoms leading to the diagnosis of an OSAS. In prevalence studies of SDB, AHI often is addressed independently of associated symptoms or the cardiovascular risk. As more and more people have been screened for possible SDB in recent years, due to more widely applicable diagnostic tools, increasing prevalence rates are shown when focusing only on the AHI. In 1993, the first systematic study on the prevalence of SDB reported 4% in men and 2% in women.[2] A meta-analysis by Peppard and colleagues[1] showed that 10% of men and 3% of women, ages 30 years to 49 years, and 17% of men and 9% of women, between the ages of 50 years and 70 years, suffered from OSA, as defined by an AHI of greater than or equal to 15 events/h. This study also showed an increase in prevalence over the past 2 decades and, furthermore, an increase with subject age. The HypnoLaus study,[3] a large epidemiologic cohort study in Switzerland, indicated a prevalence of 49% in men and 23% in women for persons over 40 years of age based on an AHI of at least 15/h. The German Study of Health in Pomerania study revealed comparable results.[4]

When deciding whether SDB should be treated, AHI severity grade, associated symptoms, and an existing risk profile (eg, cardiovascular comorbidities) are taken into account. Whether individuals with a diagnosis of SDB based on AHI without any symptoms have health consequences needs to be investigated in future epidemiologic studies. There may be a type of sleep apnea that does no harm to the cardiovascular system and could be a sign of aging. Poor sleep also can be related to complaints of insomnia with too short or fragmented sleep, movements during sleep, or having enough sleep but not being refreshed. Therefore, valid methods for diagnostics in the home environment are of great importance, allowing physicians to assess the severity of a potential sleep-related disorder. Severity should take into account not only the number and duration of apnea and hypopnea events and low oxygen saturation value events in terms of number and desaturation but also individual symptoms and risk profile. The assessment of individual consequences, however, of an existing SDB has not been well defined until now.

PART I: DIAGNOSTICS OF SLEEP-DISORDERED BREATHING
Challenges for Sleep Measurement in the Home-based Setting

Epidemiologic studies suggest that the prevalence of SDB exceeds the original estimate.[3] Among the participants, there are a large number of undiagnosed patients, including those with severe graded OSA according to AHI. This is of particular concern because recent studies suggest an association between OSA and increased cardiovascular risk as well as increased general health risk compared with control subjects, snorers, or patients with controlled SDB. In contrast, in patients with asymptomatic SDB receiving continuous positive airway pressure (CPAP), no positive effect on cardiovascular mortality could be shown.[5,6] This is opposed by the fact that positive airway pressure (PAP) therapy significantly reduced snoring and observed daytime sleepiness and improved subjective quality of life in treated patients. It can be concluded that the AHI does not seem to be a suitable parameter for identifying patients at cardiovascular risk. Additionally, recent studies show that SDB severity in patients shows a considerable night-to-night variability, suggesting that a 1-night measurement is not appropriate to estimate SDB severity.[7]

Telemedical Methods in Sleep Medicine

With technological evolution, development of medicine also has made great strides toward personalized medicine, including the application of telemedical approaches. Various studies have shown the benefits of telemedical applications in terms of patient-centered medicine, reduction of costs, and increasing access to medical care for patients with chronic diseases, especially in underserved or rural areas as well as in low-income countries.[8–12]

Most telemedical applications are used for long-term management of chronic diseases or therapy control rather than for diagnostics. Thus, the area of telemedicine in sleep medicine often is regarded as a focused and limited application field for telemedicine technologies covering only a small amount of telemedicine, which is defined as "the use of electronic information and communication technologies to provide and support health care when distance separates patient and health care unit or professional"[13–15] by the means of all kinds of tele-communication tools, including smartphones, wire-less devices for out-of-center (OOC) testing,[16] and video and telephone consultations.

Aspects of telemedicine that are relevant for sleep medicine include the wireless recording of sleep and vital functions during sleep, wireless recording of respiration, wireless data transmis-sion for recorded data, assessment of sleep and sleep apnea using smartphone technologies, and telemedical monitoring of therapy compliance in SDB patients.

Telesleep Medicine

Given the limited resource of diagnostic gold stan-dard of polysomnography (PSG) and the even more limited resource of sleep physicians, telemedicine strategies could contribute to a more comprehen-sive sleep medicine care. Through telediagnostics at locations without sleep medicine care, the sleep medicine care network could be expanded. Video consultation especially, which had been pushed by COVID-19 pandemic, could bring affected pa-tients to a suitable sleep medicine expertise at an early stage. Teletherapy also would be conceivable through digital connections between care units. Teleconsultation between treating physicians could be helpful, especially in view of the interdisciplinary nature of the complaints and comorbidities in sleep apnea. Corresponding recommendations for the establishment of telemedical approaches in sleep medicine practice recently were published by the American Academy of Sleep Medicine (AASM).[17] The technologies are available today and can be implemented as part of a sleep medicine care concept. In addition to the lack of infrastructure, there is a lack of appreciation of the topic of sleep and sleep medicine among payers and health pol-icy makers. This is surprising when considering the economic consequences caused by sleep disorders.

Out-of-Center Sleep Measurement

Technical developments in the field of diagnostics can be differentiated according to type of recording and evaluation of sleep, type of sensor technology, and use of telemedicine applications. Ambulatory devices could be beneficial additions to the already existing patient pathway, because they are suited for long-term use. In contrast to 1-night PSG measurements in the sleep labora-tory, OOC devices are able to determine night-to-night variability in SDB severity.

Furthermore, the usage of wearables, devices, and apps for long-term monitoring is adapted for more distinct patient empowerment. This could be an important step to improved long-term compliance.

The high prevalence of SDB has been the best trigger for the development and application of portable devices for home-based sleep testing during the past decades. These devices are cut down to the most relevant variables (ie, estimation of sleep and wakefulness, oronasal airflow, respi-ratory effort, oxygen saturation, and body posi-tion).[18–22] Recent portable sleep apnea testing devices have gained increasing diagnostic accu-racy compared with the reference standard PSG.

Most systems allow the application of sensors by patients themselves in a home-based setting after clarification by a member of the sleep medi-cine centers. In most centers, the evaluation is semivisual. Continuous improvement of the algo-rithms on which evaluations are based will keep sleep researchers busy for many years.

Some systems need patients to enter sleep times manually, for example, lights off for intended sleep onset and lights on for intended wake-up time, for software valuation reasons. All of these portable systems are called home sleep apnea testing (HSAT), polygraphy, or OOC devices.[16,19–21] HSAT is limited to SDB assessment at home. The term, polygraphy, is a synonym often used in Europe. OOC includes HSAT and the term is broader, covering many implementations, because it mentions and defines sleep recording as well. Different OOC levels define different accuracy, for example for sleep, from home PSG on the top down to actigraphy as a simple assessment device for sleep.

Preserving Traditions: Established Techniques and Further Developments

A diagnosis of SDB follows a stepwise approach, starting with the family physician and out-patient service moving up to an interdisciplinary sleep medicine center with all diagnostic options avail-able. First is assessment of complaints about un-restful sleep that needs to quantify how long this has been the case. Then, symptoms of sleepiness, initiating sleep, maintaining sleep, and impact on social and work life need to be assessed. The sec-ond step is an assessment of sleepiness with vali-dated questionnaires, possibly cardiopulmonary testing, or cognitive testing. The third step is an OOC recording for SDB if this is suspected. If the HSAT does not provide a clarification of com-plaints and symptoms, a fourth step is required, which is cardiorespiratory PSG under supervision of trained staff. The availability of supervised PSG is limited and costs are high.

In order to evaluate and categorize systems available for HSAT, recently a scheme had been proposed. The categorization system is based on an assessment of the monitored physiologic functions.[16] It categorizes OOC devices based on recordings of sleep, cardiovascular, oximetry, position, effort, and respiratory (SCOPER) parameters. Categorization then is based on the number of electroencephalogram (EEG) electrodes used for sleep measurement, the number of electrocardiography (ECG) leads and respiratory inductive plethysmography belts, the type of body position determination (eg, use of video recording), and the type of respiration measurement (thermistor or nasal cannula). New OOC devices for SDB estimation, however, that use parameters according to SCOPER also must be certified according to the Medical Devices Act and validated against the reference PSG in order to prove clinical applicability.

Actigraphy and Accelerometry

Actigraphy and accelerometry measurements are noninvasive methods for monitoring activity and rest cycles. They are suitable for use in large collectives for activity determination as well as for sleep monitoring.[23] They offer an affordable, user-friendly, and scalable alternative to PSG to monitor sleep-wake cycles and now are recognized by the AASM as a valid method for sleep assessment.[24] Recent advances in artificial intelligence and larger studies in conjunction with PSG are leading to steady improvements in the methodology.

However, 3 key limitations of actigraphy and accelerometry remain. There is a lack of validation studies for the different lifestyle devices. Standardization of approaches for human activity recognition is missing. And, finally, assessment of daytime naps using actigraphy needs to be discussed critically.[25] Currently, wearables often are used combined with other minimally invasive sensors to gain more health-related data.

Electronic Health and Mobile Health in Respiratory Sleep Medicine

Novel methods from the fields of electronic health (e-health) and mobile health (m-health) offer smart solutions for problems that currently still are insufficiently addressed.

Determining the pretest probability is crucial for targeted diagnostic and therapeutic strategies for OSA. Today, apps already provide users with validated digital screening methods. One such screening tool is the NoSAS (neck circumference, obesity, snoring, age, and sex) score, which has been validated in studies.[26] The NoSAS score, which ranges from 0 to 17, includes 5 questions: 4 points for a neck circumference greater than 40 cm, 3 points for a body mass index (BMI) of 25 kg/m^2 to less than 30 kg/m^2 or 5 points for a BMI of 30 kg/m^2 or greater, 2 points for complained snoring, 4 points for age 55 years, and 2 points for male gender. The NoSAS score identifies individuals at risk of clinically significant SDB at a threshold of 8 points. The STOP-BANG (the snoring, tiredness, observed apnea, high blood pressure, BMI, age, neck circumference, and male gender) score, another validated screening questionnaire to determine the likelihood of OSA, also is available online (STOP-BANG tool Web site: http://www.stopbang.ca/).

Smartphones offer a wide range of sensors, for example, gyroscopes, microphones, and accelerometers,[27] which can be used to monitor sleep patterns. For instance, the commercial app iSleep[28] leverages a smartphone's built-in microphone to detect respiratory events like cough and snoring or body movements by processing the acoustic signals with an accuracy of greater than 90% for event classification (snoring, cough, and sleep). An important limitation of the system is that this microphone sampling represents a significant source of battery power consumption. Several other sleep apps can be purchased using various app stores. Sleep Cycle[29] is one of the most popular apps, based on both accelerometry and microphone techniques to track sleep and provide personalized alarm clocks, waking up the users during light sleep.

In addition, a wide range of wearable smartwatches and activity bands have been developed to estimate sleep. These devices often derive their metrics using a combination of movement signals (accelerometry, as discussed previously) and heart rate and heart rate variability. Various studies assess the validation or reliability of some of the most common brands on the measurement of physical activity and sleep (Fitbit, Garmin, Misfit, Apple, Polar, and Samsung).

Other apps try to detect breathing disorders during sleep using sensors integrated in the smartphone. They use microphones or acceleration sensors or even turn the smartphone into an active sonar system that emits frequency-modulated sound signals and detects their reflections. In this way, respiration-dependent movements of the thorax and abdomen can be inferred and sleep apnea episodes identified. To improve the significance, additional sensors can be coupled with an app on the smartphone—measuring strips or activity mats that are placed under the mattress or bed frame or contactless radar measuring devices that measure body movements during sleep and thus can infer the presence of sleep apnea.

Bed and Mattress Sensors

Bed and mattress sensors are defined as a sensor monitoring physiologic processes like respiration or heart rate while being placed on the bed. Mostly these devices are based on the piezoelectric effect or ballistocardiography signal recording.[30–32] One recent example is the commercially available home sleep monitoring device, Beddit Sleep Monitor,[33] a thin strip sensor that is placed under the mattress topper. The Beddit Sleep Monitor is a 3-channel movement detection sensor, which originally was designed as a substitute for the static charge sensitive bed sensor. The Beddit Sleep Monitor transmits body, respiratory, and heart movement data via a Bluetooth connection to a commercially designed app to calculate sleep parameters. An automated algorithm then transforms these aggregated sleep measures into a graph, compares it to previous nights, and provides information about sleep parameters in a cloud service. Withings takes the same approach with its Sleep Analyzer 2 (https://www.withings.com/de/de/store?gclsrc=aw.ds&gclid=CjwKCAjw4KyJBhAbEiwAaAQbEzEdrdFAos1Z2tnV1jHypOnd1I90feqUv-6k4SI9gk_qRyU9D6MbkhoC6KsQAvD_BwE). Nevertheless, a range of determinants can influence the performance of these methods, from postural differences to intersubject variability in BMI and preexisting clinical conditions.

Low-contact, Self-applicable Electroencephalography Diagnostics

Electroencephalography (EEG) is 1 of the most important components of the reference PSG and is used in neuropsychiatric tests and applications. Sleep EEG requires setup by an experienced technician and can be uncomfortable for the patient. In addition, it is not portable and, therefore, not suitable for home recording. Several established companies and start-ups are been trying to establish wireless EEGs in the sleep medicine market for the past decade. The performance of the launched systems has been compared with conventional sleep EEG with strong correlations.[34,35] A study of Koley and colleagues[36] showed that automatic scoring using ensemble models on a single-channel EEG reached a strong correlation coefficient r = 0.87 compared with visual scoring in clinical environment.

Recordings of the EEG signal with new miniaturized sensors inside the ear channel, so-called "in-ear EEG" sensors are a modality that has shown promise in recent years. A study by Mikkelsen and colleagues[37] investigated a machine learning (ML)-based sleep-wake staging method using data from a self-applicable electroencephalogram (cEEGrid) in addition to actigraphy in 15 healthy persons. The comparison with the visual evaluation showed that the method is equivalent to other automatic evaluation algorithms. They found a good intraclass correlation coefficient (ICC) for TST (total sleep time) (ICC = 0.82) but only a moderate ICC for SE (sleep efficacy) and REM (rapid eye movement) latency (ICC = 0.47 and ICC = 0.01, respectively). Also, Nox medical (Reykjavik, Iceland) provides a self-applicable EEG for performing PSG in patients' home environment for research purposes (https://noxmedical.com/about/news-press/article/nox-research-presents-3-abstracts-at-world-sleep-2019/).

Ultrasound Sensors

Ultrasound sensors recently have been used to detect body movement and breathing in sleeping subjects. These sensors provide information regarding the frequency and type of body movement based on the Doppler effect.[32,38,39] This technique is comparable to radar systems (discussed later) and allows the retrieval of parameters related to breathing rate, heart rate, and body motion, with an 86% accuracy and negligible bias. Limitations of this method are the fine adjustment required based on the type of targeted body and the sensitivity to small movements.[40]

Radiofrequency-based Sensors—WiFi and Radio Signal Techniques

Radar, microwave, and radiofrequency technologies are used often in automotive industry for distance estimation. Recently, these technologies demonstrated their ability to quantify body movements with a precision allowing estimating physiologic signals causing tiny skin wall movements, such as heart beat, respiration, and movements. Devices exploit the Doppler effect by emitting a low-energy radio wave toward the patient in bed and then detecting the phase difference between the emitted and the reflected signal from the patient.[41–43]

By using artificial intelligence techniques, it is possible to determine breathing patterns, heart rate, and full-body motion. These biological signals also can be used to estimate sleep stages. The main challenge with this approach is that the signal is noisy and the information related to sleep needs to be extracted, which requires good filters. Additionally, the measurement conditions are strongly dependent on the patients being monitored. For example, in patients with sleep-related movement disorders, estimation of sleep-related parameters by this technique is difficult because the underlying algorithm misclassifies the movement-rich epochs as awake.

Examples of devices based on the WiFi signal technique are the Sleepiz One (Sleepiz, Zurich, Switzerland) and the S+ (ResMed, Sydney, Australia).[44] The Sleepiz One device is placed on the bedside table or a stand beside the user's bed and points at the user's thorax from a distance of approximately 50 cm. From this position, Sleepiz One transmits a continuous electromagnetic signal at a fixed frequency, which is reflected at the user's thorax but not influenced by clothing or a blanket. The movement of the thorax relative to Sleepiz One results in phase-shifts of the reflected signal. The reflected signal then is received and preprocessed by Sleepiz One using an algorithm based on means of time series analysis[43] (Fig. 1). As part of the certification as a medical device, the Sleepiz One device currently is being compared regarding its diagnostic validity with PSG in a clinical study.

Using different filters, the sleep analytics software can extract the signals for breathing, heart beats, and body movement. Advanced algorithms then allow accurate estimation of breathing and pulse rates, detection of specific breathing patterns such as apnea events, and extraction of further sleep related features such as sleep-wake detection.

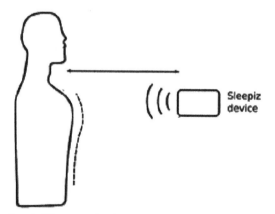

Fig. 1. Diagram of radar operation. Transmitted electromagnetic signal is reflected on the body, due to movements of the body (breathing and heart beat) reflected waves show phase-shifts being extracted by algorithms in order to analyze vital parameters (breathing frequency, number of apneas and hypopneas, pulse rate, and heart rhythm disorders). (*Figure adapted from* McEvoy RD, Antic NA, Heeley E, et al.: CPAP for Prevention of Cardiovascular Events in Obstructive Sleep Apnea. N Engl J Med. 2016; 375(10): 919–31.)

The S+, formerly SleepMinder (BiancaMed, NovaUCD, Dublin, Ireland), also is based on this principle. Only the underlying algorithms differ. In contrast to the Sleepiz One, however, the S+ is marketed as a consumer and lifestyle product.

A wide range of different sensors now are available, based on different technologies and physical effects (Fig. 2).

Regulatory Aspects Using New Sensors for Medical Purposes

Most of these apps, however, are not validated against the diagnostic reference standard PSG. A corresponding validation, however, against established clinical diagnostics, which proves that the app really uses measures that it promises, is the basic requirement for certification as a medical device—the basis for using the app for clinical diagnostics in everyday life. The German Medical Device Directive, which will be replaced by the EU-wide Medical Device Regulation in 2021, sets high regulatory requirements depending on the risk classification sought by the manufacturer, so that a new application or technology can be used as a medical device (https://eur-lex.europa.eu/legal-content/DE/TXT/?uri=CELEX%3A32017R0745). Many manufacturers of the these applications forego such certification due to this time-consuming and personnel-intensive process as well as financial aspects, with significantly faster reimbursement of the application in the so-called lifestyle area. Well-known examples of this are, for example, the ultrasound-based sleep measurement S+ of the app SleepScore (https://www.sleepscore.com/the-science/?rfr=ssl-top-nav) and Beddit Sleep Monitor (https://www.beddit.com/), a soft strip sensor that is placed on the mattress. Other providers deliberately opt for the certification process as a medical device. Current examples include integrated pulse oximeters in smartwatches and fitness trackers from Apple or Withings (https://www.imore.com/ces-2020-withings-new-smartwatch-can-help-detect-sleep-apnea) for diagnosing nocturnal oxygen desaturations as an indication of previously undetected sleep apnea. As soon as such a feature is officially certified as a medical device, however, this means that treating physicians should react clinically to pathologic measured values: for example, further diagnostics then could be initiated. For example, the ECG function of the Apple Watch already is being used in cardiologic atrial fibrillation diagnostics.[45] New contactless infrared camera technology also currently is being tested in clinical trials against the diagnostic gold standard PSG with the aim of certification as a medical device.

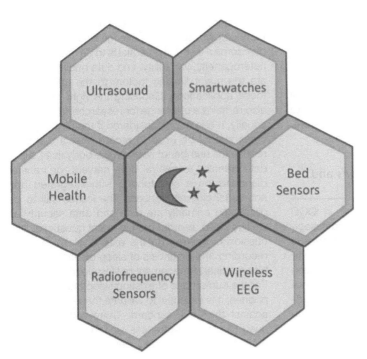

Fig. 2. Current sleep sensing technologies. (*Adapted from* Perez-Pozuelo I, Zhai B, Palotti J, Mall R, Aupetit M, Garcia-Gomez JM, Taheri S, Guan Y, Fernandez-Luque L. The future of sleep health: a data-driven revolution in sleep science and medicine. NPJ Digit Med. 2020 Mar 23; 3:42.)

Big Data and Data Science

All these questions and requirements can be addressed adequately only if the large amounts of data (also known as big data) that are collected every night in sleep laboratories are analyzed for previously unrecognized information, correlations, or patterns using novel methods of clinical data science and examined for their clinical significance.[18] These findings are not intended, however, to replace the human, medical art of healing, but to support the treating physicians in their decision making. More capacity also could be created by freeing up time resources through optimized processes.

Novel, low-contact sensor technology also enables longer-term sleep diagnostics in the home over weeks and months; thus, on the 1 hand, the investigation of the dynamics of sleep-related respiratory disorders, and, on the other hand, a clearer assessment of the actual disease burden of the patients. Established sleep laboratory examinations only allow looking at a few examination nights—but the night-to-night variability of sleep apnea seems to be of too little importance, especially in cardiologic patients. Linz and colleagues[7] were able to show that patients with paroxysmal atrial fibrillation had a clear dynamic in the degree of sleep apnea, which correlated significantly with the atrial fibrillation load during the day. Something similar is known,

for example, in dialysis patients. Big data also means, that keeping track of the data volumes is hardly possible. There is an increasing need to use computer-based analysis methods. These include self-learning algorithms. Unfortunately, their results are no longer transparent to humans. Interdisciplinary teamwork, therefore, is becoming increasingly important, because (sleep) physicians are not necessarily computer scientists or data scientists at the same time. Even sleep medicine data alone do not form uniform pictures of patients. The holistic approach, therefore, includes the integration of other clinical data and also data from patients' everyday lives. Ideally, these data should be integrated and analyzed, taking into account their interaction—a long-term goal that seems feasible only through the definition of uniform data formats and interface standards, that is, a true telematics infrastructure.

Data Sovereignty, Data Protection, and Digital Ethics

Despite all the future promises that such data aggregation and integration hold, not only for (respiratory) sleep medicine, one thing should not be forgotten: patients are and remain the masters of their data. The EU-wide General Data Protection Regulation not only is intended to minimize the risk of data misuse but also requires a declaration of consent by the patient prior to any data use, which also must be revocable at any time.[19] A revocation or nonconsent also should not lead to a disadvantage of a patient. This applies just as much to consent to data use—because there should be awareness of 1 thing: the primary goal of digitalization in health care should continue to be the well-being of the patients. This, therefore, also requires a rethinking of digital ethics.

Where To Go from Here? Conclusions and Perspectives

A more accurate diagnostic approach in OOC testing[16] could reduce invested efforts and associated costs significantly. Hence, smarter diagnostic devices integrating automatic data processing algorithms could enable a more accurate detection of SDB in the home setting without a time-consuming, personnel-consuming, and cost-consuming PSG examination. Certainly, in the future, PSG still will be an essential technology, especially for patients with complex comorbidities. New diagnostic approaches could lead to a more efficient utilization of existing sleep laboratory capacities for patients desperately requiring those resources, because current waiting time for a PSG examination is long: for example, approximately 4 months on average in Germany.[46,47] An increase of the diagnostic accuracy of OOC testing by improved diagnostic techniques compared with gold standard PSG could help to narrow the gap between the high prevalence of SDB and current limited diagnostic capacities.

Additionally, patients with sleep apnea or other sleep-related diseases have different phenotypes, individual needs, preferences, and attitudes that can have a significant impact on treatment decisions. Therefore, the use of OOC devices is necessary and desirable. As technology advances, the amount of clinical data resources available to biomedical research continues to grow.[48] Clinical data resources include open-source data from e-health medical records, medical image databases, genomic archives, and data generated by commercial applications.[48–50] Currently, sleep data repositories, such as Sleepdata.org, are being created to drive research. These databases include multimodal sleep data of all recording modalities, such as PSG to actigraphy and questionnaires, and an aim to create benchmarks for ML technologies. These developments are critical for creating valid ML models for clinical and commercial application to further understanding of the role of sleep in quality of life and morbidity.[51] Sleep-related technologies not only are useful for diagnostics but also can be used to monitor therapy and increase

compliance. Despite the high potential of these technologies, several challenges still need to be overcome if their full potential is to be realized. Their heterogeneity, variability, and data quality currently are the major limiting factors to the efficiency of these applications. Choosing the right algorithms also remains a challenge for researchers.[52,53] Additionally, it has to be considered if the new technologies should be used to record over a distance, reduce the number of wires on the body itself, allow data transfer to central data servers, or transfer diagnosis on a smartphone with integrated and additional external sensors. The issues still to be discussed primarily are data and data security as well as sleep disorder management questions. Discussion is needed on the extent to which sleep recording and diagnosis of sleep disorders constitute medical management or lifestyle management. For the current use of existing sleep apps in smartphones, it is essential to validate these applications against the gold standard. There also is a great need to spread awareness among physicians and patients on the potential benefits and limitations

Table 1
Smart diagnostics of sleep-disordered breathing

Opportunities	Risks
Precision medicine	Culture of innovation—data security/data heritage/data sovereignty
Patient-centered medicine	Data silos
Quality assurance/ improvement	Data quality
Big data analytics	Overestimation of statistical relevance in data evaluation
Trajectories	General conditions
ML/AI	Dependence on technical infrastructure
Drug monitoring/	Investment in industrialization of medicine
Patient safety	Cultural change
Efficiency improvement	Unequal participation if not equipped with digital devices
	Unequal participation with low digital literacy

Opportunities versus risks.

of sleep apps and related data sovereignty as they become available.

To achieve maximum benefit for the end user and other stakeholders (eg, hospitals, researchers, healthcare authorities, and industry), there is an increasing need for a privacy-secure and effective clinical biomarker ecosystem with algorithmic transparency, interoperable components and sensors, and open interfaces that enable high integrity of measurement systems (**Table 1**).

PART II: SMART THERAPY STRATEGIES IN SLEEP-DISORDERED BREATHING
Therapy Strategies for Sleep-disordered Breathing Using Digital Tools

The therapy for sleep-related breathing disorders is the domain of medical aids, because only a small proportion of patients can be treated by surgical therapy, and obesity, which often is at least partly responsible, in addition to age and anatomic changes, unfortunately can be treated successfully only in the long term in a few cases. Assistive therapy shares the challenge of drug therapy— adherence to therapy is of decisive importance in order to achieve the set therapy goals.

Therapy for OSA is the main task of respiratory sleep medicine. Primarily, CPAP or automatic variation of continuous positive airway pressure (APAP) therapy is used.[14] Therapeutic alternatives are mandibular advancement splints, positional therapies with positioning aids, and hypoglossal nerve stimulation, depending on degree of severity and a patient's risk profile. All therapies aim to prevent nocturnal breathing disorders and their consequences by keeping the upper airway open. The therapies are highly effective if they are applied precisely, whereby it is true for all therapies that the success of the therapy depends both on the adherence to the therapy in the sense of daily application and on the intensity of the application, that is, the duration of application during sleep.[54,55] This is due to the fact that on 1 hand there is a dose-response effect: the more intensive the use, the better the effect on, for example, symptoms or blood pressure. On the other hand, the effect of the therapy quickly is lost during breaks in therapy.[56,57] Despite many technical developments in therapy, adherence to CPAP therapy for OSA, for example, has not improved, as a recently published meta-analysis shows.[58] Exact figures are not available but it can be assumed that more than 90% of patients with OSA in German sleep laboratories are treated primarily with CPAP/APAP therapy. Therefore, the main focus in the following discussion is on this therapy.

Digital technologies are tools that should be meaningfully integrated into care processes to support them. Telemonitoring as a remote transmission of therapy data without defined actions triggered by these data does not bring any relevant benefit on its own. Telemonitoring data must be used to identify the right patients who need support. Furthermore, the transmitted data must be included in an appropriate care structure. Therefore, it is important to consider the telemedicine methodology, especially the type of intervention, in all studies. Ultimately, data can ever be transformed into beneficial outcomes only through human expertise—only if telemedicine additively supports the medical decision-making process in this way will it benefit patients.

Therapy Adherence Through Participation

As demanded in precision medicine approaches, patients should be actively involved in their therapy and be able to participate in it (patient engagement). Patients receive feedback that can give them important support in achieving both therapy adherence and therapy quality, especially in the critical early phase of therapy. The first systems of this kind already are available (eg, DreamMapper, Philips Respironics [Murrysville, Pennsylvania]; myAir, ResMed [San Diego, California]). In the absence of randomized trials on the use of these systems, various analyses of therapy device data indicate that the use of such a patient engagement system is associated with significantly more intensive use of PAP therapy.[59] An analysis of the first 500 patients in Germany supported by a patient engagement system (MyAir) shows a relevantly higher use of PAP therapy when using the feedback system compared with a cohort with statistical twins (matching).[60]

Although long-term adherence often is determined in the first 14 days of PAP therapy, follow-up usually is after 6 weeks to 12 weeks.[61] An outpatient clinical control is planned—possibly with the use of an additional outpatient polygraphy. Furthermore, annual controls are recommended.[14] Even at this early stage, therapy adherence can be objectified by using the therapy device data. In addition to therapy adherence, therapy can be optimized through further data from the therapy device: thus, estimates of therapy quality often are possible based on the data provided. Depending on the device manufacturer, application duration, application frequency, respiratory disturbances total/differentiated, leakage, humidifier application, and pressure curve are available, although no uniform validation is available for almost all of this information. Furthermore, for some devices, no validation data are published at all. The problem for the colleagues providing follow-up care is that each device requires its own software. In addition, the effort for reading out the therapy device is not remunerated. Here, digitalization through telemedicine can make an important contribution to structural care. It must also be fundamentally clarified who is responsible for which aspects of therapeutic care. Currently, health insurance companies conclude contracts with homecare providers that give the providers responsibility for achieving sufficient therapy adherence. In addition to clarifying the medical definition, the remuneration also must be adjusted.

Clinical Study Situation: Telemedical Therapy Monitoring in Obstructive Sleep Apnea

Although the care situation continues to need clarification, there is growing evidence in recent years on the use of telemedicine in the context of PAP therapy for OSA. It is important to consider the telemedicine methodology, type of intervention, and targeting criteria in all studies conducted.

The first large randomized trial in 2010 using automated telephone feedback in 250 patients with newly diagnosed OSA showed a median increase in CPAP use in the intervention group of 0.9 h/night at 6 months and 2.0 h/night at 12 months after 12 months of telemedicine intervention.[62] The motivational interviewing technique was used. Motivational interviewing is a pragmatic concept of interviewing in order to win people over for change. In 2012, a randomized trial compared proactive patient care supported by telemonitoring with conventional therapy initiation in the sleep laboratory.[63] The data transmitted by the PAP therapy device were reviewed regularly and patients were contacted by telephone if there were any abnormalities (poor use, high leakage, increased residual respiratory disturbances, and high therapy pressure). Therapy problems and associated complaints were queried and a targeted intervention, such as a mask change, was arranged. In the telemedicine arm, there was a significant increase in therapy use after 3 months, both in terms of average daily use and in terms of use on days when therapy was applied. The study was relatively small, with 75 patients, so that other endpoints regarding therapy effectiveness showed a trend toward improvement, but this was not statistically significant due to the small number of cases. A German publication compared the therapy discontinuation rate after 1 year in patients who were proactively supported by their homecare provider through telemonitoring with conventional reactive care (**Fig. 3**).[64] Proactive

means that the therapy device data (use and leakage) available via telemonitoring were checked regularly. In cases of poor therapy use, patients were contacted, therapy problems were queried in a standardized way, and possible solutions, for example, intensification of humidification or mask change, were pointed out. In contrast, with traditional reactive care, patients had to report therapy problems independently to the homecare provider or to their sleep laboratory. Proactive care was associated with a halving of the treatment discontinuation rate (therapy termination rate at 1 year follow-up, 11.0% vs 5.4%, respectively; $P<.001$).[64] This also was seen in the subgroups studied (men/women, type of health insurance, and type of PAP therapy). This was not a randomized study, however, but a comparison of 2 groups from health care reality. The selection bias of group comparisons was minimized through targeted matching, and large groups were compared (3401 patients per group).

A randomized trial from France attempted to improve blood pressure control in patients with OSA on nocturnal CPAP therapy by using a more complex telemedicine intervention.[65] Patients were required to document PAP therapy and blood pressure data via a smartphone and received daily nutrition and physical activity pictograms as support. Both groups received intensive support regarding their CPAP therapy with a telephone visit after 2 days and a sleep medical check-up after 4 weeks. Both arms showed good, comparable adherence to PAP therapy and no difference in measured blood pressure at home. Another recent randomized trial of 206 patients using a telemedicine-based care strategy in patients at low cardiovascular risk also failed to show an improvement in treatment adherence.[66] In a Spanish randomized trial of telemonitoring in 100 newly diagnosed OSA patients on PAP therapy, there was no difference in treatment adherence and treatment effect in either arm with good treatment adherence. Although the telemedicine approach saved costs, patient satisfaction was greater during face-to-face follow-up.[67] The Spanish sleep apnea working group used a different telemedicine approach in their research project.[68] They developed a Web site for patients with disease and therapy information, where the course of therapy was documented by the patient. The documented data were monitored by the sleep laboratory, and the sleep laboratory could communicate with the patient via the Web site. In addition, video visits were conducted via the Web site using Skype after 1 month and 3 months. The clinical outcomes were comparable and the telemedicine approach was cost-effective. The

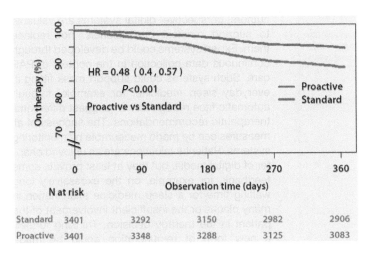

Fig. 3. Kaplan-Meier plot: PAP therapy discontinuation rate in patients with proactive therapy monitoring using telemonitoring (Proactive) compared with standard care (Standard). HR, hazard ratio. (*From* Woehrle H, Ficker JH, Graml A, et al. Telemedicine-based proactive patient management during positive airway pressure therapy: Impact on therapy termination rate. Somnologie 2017; 21: 121-127.)

N at risk					
Standard	3401	3292	3150	2982	2906
Proactive	3401	3348	3288	3125	3083

telemedicine approach reduced indirect costs (lost work time and travel costs to the sleep laboratory). Other studies in different health systems showed a reduction in work for the nurses and the sleep laboratory, respectively, and a faster intervention.[69–71] The largest and also a very complex study on the use of telemedicine options in 1455 patients with suspected OSA compared the additional use of Web-based patient education and the use of telemonitoring of PAP therapy with an automated feedback system via email, SMS, or phone calls.[72] The telemedicine-based patient feedback led to an improvement in treatment adherence after 90 days, whereas the additional patient education had no effect on this. There was only a sustained improvement in adherence over time when telemedicine-assisted patient feedback was continued. A Japanese study investigated the benefit of telemedicine-supported follow-up for PAP therapy that already had been established for 1 month for noninferiority compared with the current, very costly, face-to-face follow-up. Noninferiority of the telemedicine approach was shown.[73]

Initial feasibility data for telemedical adherence management in the context of mandibular advancement splint therapy show good approaches and also should be established firmly in the management of this increasingly important therapy for OSA. Similar approaches exist for tongue pacemaker therapy and also should be pursued further.

Telemedicine-assisted Positive Airway Pressure Initiation?

An additional, specific aspect of telemedicine for sleep medicine care is the potential enabling of PAP therapy initiation outside the sleep laboratory. PSG, which is performed routinely in Germany and used to prescribe a PAP therapy device, is not mandatory in patients without significant comorbidities (eg, relevant heart failure or chronic obstructive pulmonary disease) when looking at the available evidence internationally. Several studies, also from recent years, show no advantage here for PSG-monitored therapy initiation.[74,75] By including telemonitoring, the initial phase of therapy can be accompanied more intensively, whereby the handling of the data and the clinical consequences drawn from it also are decisive. In a comparability study recently completed in Germany between PSG-assisted therapy initiation and outpatient therapy initiation supported by telemonitoring, no difference was shown after 6 months with regard to therapy adherence and the therapy effect on sleep apnea symptoms and quality of life.[76]

Precision Medicine Through telemedicine

Another new aspect of continuous follow-up is the concept of trajectories (movement paths) of monitored parameters. Current clinical strategies are based on single, day-by-day analyses of mostly polygraphic follow-up. At least in the follow-up of CPAP/APAP therapy, initial analyses of large data sets of PAP therapy devices show that the continuously recorded trajectory of an elevated central apnea index better reflects the clinical value of the central apnea load than that of a single night. Using data from more than 130,000 therapy devices analyzed,[77] it was shown that CSA initially occurred in 3.5% of patients on CPAP/APAP therapy but regressed within the first 3 months in 55% of patients (transient CSA) (**Fig. 4**). CSA persisted in 25% of patients (persistent CSA), whereas CSA developed in 20% of patients (emerging CSA). Another analysis of the therapy device database looked at the change in therapy from CPAP/APAP therapy to adaptive servo-ventilation

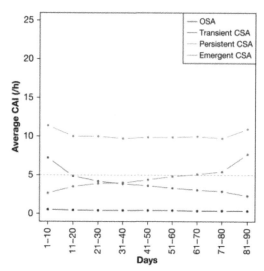

Fig. 4. Trajectories regarding the development of CSA phases (CAI) under nocturnal CPAP therapy in patients with OSA, transient CSA, persistent CSA, and emergent CSA. CAI, central apnea index. (*From* Liu D, Armitstead J, Benjafield A, et al. Trajectories of Emergent Central Sleep Apnea During CPAP Therapy. Chest 2017; 152: 751-760)

therapy in patients with persistent CSA (see **Fig. 4**).[77] It was shown that the change in therapy had the expected therapeutic effect of significantly improved control of respiratory disorders. The switch to adaptive servo-ventilation also was associated with a stabilization of therapy utilization at a high level, after a continuous deterioration under CPAP/APAP.

Perspective

Digital technologies are tools that should be meaningfully integrated into care processes to support them. Telemonitoring alone does not make anything better. The monitoring data must be used to identify the right patients who need support in order to include them in an appropriate care structure. In this context, it is important to develop systems that can also visualize a large number of patients in a manageable way (cockpit/patient dashboard).

From the authors' point of view, the study situation can be considered positive despite its inhomogeneity. The inclusion of digital/telemedical technologies in the follow-up of a PAP therapy enables the implementation of continuous, uniform, scalable, and high-quality patient care. Patient participation in their therapy through patient engagement systems can establish an important part of modern precision medicine. From the

authors' perspective, digital systems are valuable to support medical professionals, not replace them. Expert systems could be developed through continuous data collection in the context of PAP care. Such systems could support mask fitting in everyday sleep medicine, for example, through automatic face recognition, or suggest differential therapeutic recommendations. The success of all measures can be made measurable by monitoring systems. Patient evaluations are an unloved chapter of digital media, but they at least provide some feedback, for example, on the excessively long waiting time for a sleep medicine examination in many places or the insufficient involvement of the patient in the therapy decision. Thinking further, a new form of remuneration could be made possible by objectifying the success of the therapy. A so-called pay-for-performance model could enable a more success-oriented payment for sleep medicine as well as for medical technology companies. The challenge, however, is the setting of defined therapy goals and their linkage to remuneration. The experiences in medicine of the last decades show that innovations prevail in the long term only if suitable remuneration structures also are created.

Vision

The moonshot of respiratory sleep medicine is an automated patient care system, OSA—autopilot, which uses e-health and m-health to detect sleep apnea at an early stage; treats it precisely, holistically, and adaptively as well as taking into account its risk constellation; and involves patients by integrating their preferences. Such systems already would be technically feasible today if the corresponding data were available. It will be important not only to observe these developments but also to actively shape the development and the framework conditions to ensure that the care of patients with sleep-related respiratory disorders remain a medical domain. Otherwise, the door will be opened to the outsourcing of specialist sleep medicine care to the consumer sector (as already has happened, for example, with spectacles). These integral changes also require an adaptation of the training of medical professionals to modern realities without compromising medical expertise. The image of the doctor is changing from that of a pure expert to that of a medical advisor and companion to the patient. A permanent change of the doctor-patient relationship is anticipated.

SUMMARY

Through the use of various technologies, telemedicine enables more intensive and faster care for sleep apnea patients treated with PAP therapy. This can increase long-term therapy adherence as well as therapy intensity. It also can improve the success of the therapy. Not only is the use of telemedicine important but also the correct application of the data for a targeted intervention. The leading criterion seems to be the actual use of therapy. Furthermore, telemedical approaches can be used to design new care pathways, to actively involve patients in their therapy, and to reduce associated costs. Telemedicine should be a central element of modern sleep medicine care, especially in view of the high number of cases and the long waiting times for diagnostic and therapeutic interventions.

CLINICS CARE POINTS

- Any new consumer or medical device for sleep diagnostics needs to be validated against PSG. Validation studies need to be published in reviewed journals.
- New service pathways for the management of patients with SDB are developed but still need to be evaluated in terms of economics and quality regarding patient care.
- Well-approved and validated methods for diagnosing SDB are HSAT and, in cases of comorbidities, PSG.
- Digital apps can be used to treat insomnia and can be used to support therapy adherence in sleep apnea, as proved by randomized controlled trials.

FUNDING

This work was funded partially by the Russian Federation Government grant No 075 to 15 to 2019 to 1885 and funded partially by the European H2020 grant SLEEP REVOLUTION no. 965417.

ACKNOWLEDGMENTS

T. Penzel thanks Saratov State Medical University for partial support of this work.

DISCLOSURE

T. Penzel has received speaker fees from Jazz Pharma, Löwenstein Medical, and Neuwirth Medizintechnik. He has received consulting fees from Bayer Healthcare, Cerebra Inc, Jazz Pharma, and National Sleep Foundation. He owns shares of Advanced Sleep Research, The Siestagroup GmbH, and Nukute Oy. S. Dietz-Terjung reports no conflict of interest. H. Woehrle is chair of the workgroup on Digitalization of the Federal association of pneumologists in Germany and vice chair of the section sleep medicine of the German society for pneumology. He has received speaker fees and consultation fees from Astra Zeneca, Allergopharma, Bioproject, Boehringer Ingelheim, Chiesi, GSK, Novartis, Inspire, Jazz, ResMed, and Sanofi and research grants from ResMed and Novartis. C. Schöbel reports institutional research grants and institutional financial recompensation for lectures and advisory boards by AstraZeneca, Bayer, BerlinChemie, Bristol-Myers Squibb, JAZZ Pharmaceutical, Novamed, Novartis, ResMed, and Sleepiz. C. Schöbel is member of the board of German Sleep Society (DGSM) and Head of the task force Telemedicine of German Society for Internal Medicine (DGIM).

REFERENCES

1. Peppard PE, Young T, Barnet JH, et al. Increased prevalence of sleep- sleep disordered breathing in adults. Am J Epidemiol 2013;177(9):1006–14.
2. Young T, Palta M, Dempsey J, et al. The occurrence of sleep-disordered breathing among middle-aged adults. N Engl J Med 1993;328(17):1230–5.
3. Heinzer R, Vat S, Marques-Vidal P, et al. Prevalence of sleep-disordered breathing in the general population: the HypnoLaus study. Lancet Respir Med 2015;3(4):310–8.
4. Fietze I, Laharnar N, Obst A, et al. Prevalence and association analysis of obstructive sleep apnea with gender and age differences – results of SHIP-Trend. J Sleep Res 2019;28:e12770.
5. Marin JM, Carrizo SJ, Vicente E, et al. Long-term cardiovascular outcomes in men with obstructive sleep apnoea-hypopnoea with or without treatment with continuous positive airway pressure: an observational study. Lancet 2005;365(9464):1046–53.
6. McEvoy RD, Antic NA, Heeley E, et al. CPAP for prevention of cardiovascular events in obstructive sleep apnea. N Engl J Med 2016;375(10):919–31.
7. Linz D, Baumert M, Desteghe L, et al. Nightly sleep apnea severity in patients with atrial fibrillation: potential application of long-term sleep apnea monitoring. Int J Cardiol Heart Vasc 2019;24:100424.
8. Knauert M, Naik S, Gillespie MB, et al. Clinical consequences and economic costs of untreated obstructive sleep apnea syndrome. World J Otorhinolaryngol Head Neck Surg 2015;1(1):17–27.

9. Morsy NE, Farrag NS, Zaki NFW, et al. Obstructive sleep apnea: personal, societal, public health, and legal implications. Rev Environ Health 2019;34:153–69.

10. Benjafield AV, Ayas NT, Eastwood PR, et al. Estimation of the global prevalence and burden of obstructive sleep apnoea: a literature-based analysis. Lancet Respir Med 2019;7(8):687–98.

11. Wickwire EM, Tom SE, Vadlamani A, et al. Older adult US Medicare beneficiaries with untreated obstructive sleep apnea are heavier users of health care than controls. J Clin Sleep Med 2020;16:81–9.

12. Woehrle H, Arzt M, Graml A, et al. Predictors of positive airway pressure therapy termination in the first year: analysis of big data from a German homecare provider. BMC Pulm Med 2018;18:186.

13. Penzel T, Fietze I, Hirshkowitz M. Diagnostik in der Schlafmedizin. Somnologie 2011;15(2):78–83.

14. Mayer G, Arzt M, Braumann B, et al. S3-Leitlinie Nicht erholsamer Schlaf/Schlafstörungen –Kapitel "Schlafbezogene Atmungsstörungen". Somnologie 2017;20(Supplement 2):97–180.

15. Qaseem A, Dallas P, Owens DK, et al. Diagnosis of obstructive sleep apnea in adults: a clinical practice guideline from the American College of Physicians. Ann Intern Med 2014;161(3):210–20.

16. Collop NA, Tracy SL, Kapur V, et al. Obstructive sleep apnea devices for out-of-center (OOC) testing: technology evaluation. J Clin Sleep Med 2011;7(5):531–48.

17. American Academy of sleep medicine (AASM): clinical resources, telemedicine. Available at: https://aasm.org/clinical-resources/telemedicine/checkedon01.07.2020. Accessed September 27, 2021.

18. Burgdorf A, Güthe I, Jovanovic M, et al. The mobile sleep app: an open-source framework for mobile sleep assessment based on consumer-grade wearable devices. Computer Biol Med 2018;103:8–16.

19. Singh J, Badr MS, Diebert W, et al. American Academy of sleep medicine (AASM) position paper for the use of telemedicine for the diagnosis and treatment of sleep disorders. J Clin Sleep Med 2015;11(10):1187–98.

20. Randerath W, Bögel M, Franke C, et al. [Positionpaper on telemonitoring in sleep-related breathing disorders]. Pneumologie 2017;71(2):81–5.

21. Verbraecken J. Telemedicine applications in sleep disordered breathing: thinking out of the box. Sleep Med Clin 2016;11(4):445–59.

22. Ko PR, Kientz JA, Choe EK, et al. Consumer sleep technologies: a review of the landscape. J Clin Sleep Med 2015;11(12):1455–61.

23. Troiano RP, Berrigan D, Dodd KW, et al. Physical activity in the United States measured by accelerometer Med. Sci Sports Exerc 2008;40:181–8.

24. Sadeh A. The role and validity of actigraphy in sleep medicine: an update. Sleep Med Rev 2011;15:259–67.

25. Martin JL, Hakim AD. Wrist actigraphy. Chest 2011;139:1514–27.

26. Marti-Soler H, Hirotsu C, Marques-Vidal P, et al. The NoSAS score for screening of sleep-disordered breathing: a derivation and validation study. Lancet Respir Med 2016;4(9):742–8.

27. Borger JN, Huber R, Ghosh A. Capturing sleep-wake cycles by using day-today smartphone touchscreen interactions. NPJ Digital Med 2019;2:73.

28. Hao T, Xing G, Zhou G. iSleep: unobtrusive sleep quality monitoring using smartphones. Proceedings of the 11th ACM conference on embedded networked sensor systems. New York: ACM; 2013. p. 4.

29. Ong AA, Gillespie MB. Overview of smartphone applications for sleep analysis. World J Otorhinolaryngol Head Neck Surg 2016;2:45.

30. Chow P, Nagendra G, Abisheganaden J, et al. Respiratory monitoring using an air-mattress system. Physiol Meas 2000;21:345.

31. Chee Y, Han J, Youn J, et al. Air mattress sensor system with balancing tube for unconstrained measurement of respiration and heart beat movements. Physiol Meas 2005;26:413.

32. Arlotto P, Grimaldi M, Naeck R, et al. An ultrasonic contactless sensor for breathing monitoring. Sensors 2014;14:15371–86.

33. Paalasmaa J, Toivonen H, Partinen M. Adaptive heartbeat modeling for beat-to-beat heart rate measurement in ballistocardiograms. IEEE J Biomed Health Inform 2015;19(6):1945–52.

34. Kam JWY, Griffin S, Shen A, et al. Systematic comparison between a wireless EEG system with dry electrodes and a wired EEG system with wet electrodes. Neuroimage 2019;184:119–29.

35. Finan PH, Richards JM, Gamaldo CE, et al. Validation of a wireless, self-application, ambulatory electroencephalographic sleep monitoring device in healthy volunteers. J Clin Sleep Med 2016;12:1443–51.

36. Koley B, Dey D. An ensemble system for automatic sleep stage classification using single channel EEG signal. Comput Biol Med 2012;42:1186–95.

37. Mikkelsen KB, Tabar YR, Kappel SL, et al. Accurate whole-night sleep monitoring with dry-contact ear-EEG. Sci Rep 2019;9(1):16824.

38. Min SD, Yoon DJ, Yoon SW, et al. A study on a non-contacting respiration signal monitoring system using Doppler ultrasound. Med Biol Eng Comput 2007;45(11):1113–9.

39. Shahshahani, A., Bhadra, S. & Zilic, Z. A continuous respiratory monitoring system using ultrasound piezo transducer. Circuits and Systems (ISCAS), 2018 IEEE International Symposium on, 1–4 (IEEE, 2018).

40. Nijsure Y, Tay WP, Gunawan E, et al. An impulse radio ultrawideband system for contactless

noninvasive respiratory monitoring. IEEE Trans Biomed Eng 2013;60:1509–17.

41. Rahman, T. et al. DoppleSleep: a contactless unobtrusive sleep sensing system using short-range Doppler radar. Proceedings of the 2015 ACM International Joint conference on Pervasive and Ubiquitous monitoring using a single COTS TX-RX pair. Proceedings of the 13th International Symposium on Information Processing in Sensor Networks, 59–70 (IEEE Press, 2014). Berlin, April 15-17, 2014.

42. Adib F, Mao H, Kabelac Z, et al. Smart homes that monitor breathing and heart rate. in Proceedings of the 33rd annual ACM conference on human factors in computing systems. New York: ACM; 2015. p. 837–46.

43. Droitcour AD, Boric-Lubecke O, Lubecke VM, et al. Range correlation effect on ISM band I/Q CMOS radar for non-contact vital signs sensing. 2003 IEEE MTT-S international microwave Symposium digest. IEEE MTT-S International Microwave Symposium 3: vol. 3 1945 - 1948. Philadelphia, June 8-13, 2003.

44. Weinreich G, Terjung S, Wang Y, et al. Validation of SleepMinderTM as non-contact device for sleep-disordered breathing and periodic limb movement. Eur Respir J 2015;46:PA3680.

45. Perez MV, Mahaffey KW, Hedlin H, et al. Large Scale Assessment of a Smartwatch to identify atrial Fibrillation. N Engl J Med 2019;381:1909–11.

46. Available at: https://www.welt.de/regionales/thueringen/article213696506/Lange-Wartezeiten-fuer-Patienten-auf-Termin-im-Schlaflabor.html. Accessed September 27, 2021.

47. Perez-Pozuelo I, Zhai B, Palotti J, et al. The future of sleep health: a data-driven revolution in sleep science and medicine. NPJ Digit Med 2020;3:42.

48. Gewin V. Data sharing: an open mind on open data. Nature 2016;529:117–9.

49. Dinov ID. Methodological challenges and analytic opportunities for modeling and interpreting big healthcare data. Gigascience 2016;5:12.

50. Turakhia MP, Desai M, Hedlin H, et al. Rationale and design of a large-scale, app-based study to identify cardiac arrhythmias using a smartwatch: the Apple Heart Study. Am Heart J 2019;207:66–75.

51. Dean DA, Goldberger AL, Mueller R, et al. Scaling up scientific discovery in sleep medicine: the national sleep research resource. Sleep 2016;39:1151–64.

52. Sáez C, García-Gómez JM. Kinematics of big biomedical data to characterize temporal variability and seasonality of data repositories: functional data analysis of data temporal evolution over nonparametric statistical manifolds. Int J Med Inform 2018;119:109–24.

53. Sáez C, Robles M, García-Gómez JM. Stability metrics for multi-source biomedical data based on simplicial projections from probability distribution distances. Stat Methods Med Res 2017;26:312–36.

54. Schoch OD, Baty F, Niedermann J, et al. Baseline predictors of adherence to positive airway pressure therapy for sleep apnea: a 10-year single-center observational cohort study. Respiration 2014;87:121–8.

55. Weaver TE, Maislin G, Dinges DF, et al. Relationship between hours of CPAP use and achieving normal levels of sleepiness and daily functioning. Sleep 2007;30:711–9.

56. Weaver TE, Grunsteing RR. Adherence to continuous positive airway pressure therapy: the challenge to effective treatment. Proc Am Thorac Soc 2008;5:173–8.

57. Kohler M, Stoewhas AC, Ayers L, et al. Effects fo continuous positive airway pressure therapy withdrawal in patients with obstructive sleep apnea: a randomized controlled trial. Am J Respir Crit Care Med 2011;184:1192–9.

58. Rotenberg BW, Murariu D, Pang KP. Trends in CPAP adherence over twenty years of data collection: a flattened curve. J Otolaryngol 2016;45:43.

59. Malhotra A, Crocker ME, Willes L, et al. Patient engagement using new technology to improve adherence to positive airway pressure therapy: a retrospective analysis. Chest 2018;153:843–50.

60. Woehrle H, Arzt M, Graml A, et al. Effect of a patient engagement tool on positive airway pressure adherence: analysis of a German healthcare provider database. Sleep Med 2018;41:20–6.

61. Popescu G, Latham M, Allgar V, et al. Continuous positive airway pressure for sleep apnoea/hypopnoea syndrome: usefulness of a 2 week trial to identify factors associated with long term use. Thorax 2001;56:727–33.

62. Sparrow D, Aloia M, Demolles DA, et al. A telemedicine intervention to improve adherence to continuous positive airway pressure: a randomised controlled trial. Thorax 2010;65:1061–6.

63. Fox N, Hirsch-Allen AJ, Goodfellow E, et al. The impact of a telemedicine monitoring system on positive airway pressure adherence in patients with obstructive sleep apnea: a randomized controlled trial. Sleep 2012;35:477–81.

64. Woehrle H, Ficker JH, Graml A, et al. Telemedicine-based proactive patient management during positive airway pressure therapy: impact on therapy termination rate. Somnologie 2017;21:121–7.

65. Mendelson M, Vivodtzev I, Tamisier R, et al. CPAP treatment supported by telemedicine does not improve blood pressure in high cardiovascular risk OSA patients: a randomized, controlled trial. Sleep 2014;37:1863–70.

66. Tamisier R, Treptow E, Joyeux-Faure M, et al. Impact of a multimodal telemonitoring intervention on CPAP adherence in symptomatic low-cardiovascular risk

sleep apnea: a randomized controlled trial. Chest 2020;S0012–3692.

67. Turino C, de Batlle J, Woehrle H, et al. Management of continuous positive airway pressure treatment compliance using telemonitoring in obstructive sleep apnoea. Eur Respir J 2017;49:1601128.

68. Isetta V, Negrin MA, Monasterio C, et al. A Bayesian cost-effectiveness analysis of a telemedicine-based strategy for the management of sleep apnoea: a multicentre randomised controlled trial. Thorax 2015;70:1054–61.

69. Anttalainen U, Melkko S, Hakko S, et al. Telemonitoring of CPAP therapy may save nursing time. Sleep Breath 2016;20:1209–15.

70. Hoet F, Libert W, Sanida C, et al. Telemonitoring in continuous positive airway pressure-treated patients improves delay to first intervention and early compliance: a randomized trial. Sleep Med 2017;39:77–83.

71. Munafo D, Hevener W, Crocker M, et al. A telehealth program for CPAP adherence reduces labor and yields similar adherence and efficacy when compared to standard of care. Sleep Breath 2016; 20:777–85.

72. Hwang D, Chang JW, Benjafield AV, et al. Effect of telemedicine education and telemonitoring on continuous positive airway pressure adherence. The tele-OSA randomized trial. Am J Respir Crit Care Med 2018;197:117–26.

73. Murase K, Tanizawa K, Minami T, et al. A randomized controlled trial of telemedicine for long-term sleep apnea continuous positive airway pressure management. Ann Am Thorac Soc 2020; 17(3):329–37.

74. Berry RB, Sriram P. Auto-adjusting positive airway pressure treatment for sleep apnea diagnosed by home sleep testing. J Clin Sleep Med 2014;10:1269–75.

75. Corral J, Sanchez-Quiroga MA, Carmona-Bernal C, et al. Conventional polysomnography is not necessary for the management of most patients with suspected obstructive sleep apnea. Noninferiority, randomized controlled trial. Am J Respir Crit Care Med 2017;196:1181–90.

76. Lederer K, Penzel T, Lips A, et al. Randomisierte Studie zum Vergleich der Schlaflabor-gesteuerten APAP-Therapie vs. ambulant eingeleiteter Therapie bei Patienten mit OSA (DGSM conference abstract). Somnologie 2018;22(Suppl 1):1–46.

77. Liu D, Armitstead J, Benjafield A, et al. Trajectories of emergent central sleep apnea during CPAP therapy. Chest 2017;152:751–60.

Sleep Measurements in Women

Martin Ulander, PhD[a,b], Frida Rångtell, PhD[c], Jenny Theorell-Haglöw, PhD[d],*

KEYWORDS

• Objective sleep • Subjective sleep • Gender • Review • Sex differences

KEY POINTS

- Both objective and subjective measures of sleep and sleep-related variables seem to show differences between women and men.
- Most methods and instruments assessing sleep have not been substantially tested for sex or gender differences, and only few studies had the primary aim to investigate sex or gender differences.
- There are to date no guidelines as to whether or not the set up or scoring of sleep studies should be performed differently in women and men.
- Future studies need to be specifically designed to study sex or gender differences of sleep variables and focus on sex and gender differences and the interaction with age, along with possible effects of sex hormones across the life-span.

INTRODUCTION

Sleep in women and men has been investigated in several studies, showing higher prevalence of sleep complaints in women compared with men and with an increasing difference with increasing age.[1] However, polysomnography (PSG) has not clearly shown this, and some studies have also shown better objectively measured sleep in women compared with men.[2–4] In addition, chronotype has been compared between gender, showing women to be less evening type than men. However, there seems to be attenuation of this relationship with increasing age.[5]

Several factors can affect sleep, including psychological factors such as anxiety and depression. In addition, anxiety and depression have an impact on sleep and are more common in women[6,7]; this could be argued to contribute to sex differences in general sleep. Women have nonetheless been shown to be less affected by external stressors,[2] thereby arguably being less prone to stress-related sleep issues. Hormonal changes after

puberty have also been suggested as a factor contributing to sex differences in sleep seen in the adult population.[7,8] Yet another factor is age, with increasing sleep disturbances with increasing age. Nonetheless, there are some evidence that subjective sleep quality increase with increasing age in women regardless of objective measures.[9]

Because there is still a lack of knowledge on sleep measurements in women, the present review aims to produce an overview of the current knowledge of objective and subjective sleep measurements in women.

APPROACH

For this review, "sleep measurement" was defined as both objective and subjective sleep-related measurements, and we wanted to include a wide variety of measurements that are validated and used internationally. Sex and gender are terms that are often used interchangeably and have also been used interchangeably in research over the years. The term "sex" however usually

a Department of Biomedical and Clinical Sciences, Faculty of Medicine, Linkoping University, Sjukhusvägen, 581 83 Linkoping, Sweden; b Department of Clinical Neurophysiology, Linköping University Hospital, Linköping S-581 85, Sweden; c Slumra of Sweden AB, Tiundagatan 41, Uppsala 75230, Sweden; d Department of Medical Sciences, Respiratory, Allergy and Sleep Research, Uppsala University, Box 256, Uppsala 751 05, Sweden
* Corresponding author.
E-mail address: jenny.theorell-haglow@medsci.uu.se

Sleep Med Clin 16 (2021) 635–648
https://doi.org/10.1016/j.jsmc.2021.07.004

describes characteristics that are biologically defined, whereas gender is based on socially constructed features. Nonetheless, it is recognized that there are variations in how people experience gender based on self-perception and expression and how they behave. For this review, we have chosen to use both terms within the text, as different studies included in the review have used both of the terms.

We performed structured searches in the databases PubMed and Google Scholar using the following search terms: Polysomnography, Polygraphy, Actigraphy, Psychomotor Vigilance Test, Multiple Sleep Latency Test, Maintenance of Wakefulness Test, Sleep Apnea Syndromes, Sleep Wake Disorders, Sex, Gender, Women, Sleep Diary, STOP-BANG, Epworth Sleepiness Scale, Consensus Sleep Diary, Pittsburgh Sleep Diary, Pittsburgh Sleep Quality Index, Munich Chronotype Questionnaire, and Horne-Östberg Diurnal Type Scale. We also identified further studies through reference lists in already identified studies.

CURRENT EVIDENCE
Objective Measurements of Sleep and Sleep Apnea

Polysomnography, polygraphy, and actigraphy
Objective measurements of sleep include PSG, polygraphy (PG), and actigraphy. PSG is considered gold standard when assessing sleep and common sleep disorders as well as sleep-related movement disorders such as restless legs syndrome/periodic limb movement disorder, and rare sleep disorders such as narcolepsy.[10,11] PG is used for assessing sleep-related breathing disorders such as obstructive sleep apnea (OSA),[11] and actigraphy is used to record movement,[12–14] which can be further analyzed to estimate wake/sleep patterns.[12]

Several PSG studies have shown differences in objective sleep variables in women compared with men. These studies have shown longer sleep latency,[15] shorter total sleep time,[15] more slow wave sleep (SWS), and less nonrapid eye movement (NREM) sleep stage 1 and 2 in women compared with men.[16] In older adults, less delta activity (indicates so-called deep sleep) have been shown in women compared with men.[17] Also, actigraphy data have shown differences in sleep variables between women and men. However, in older adults, results have shown somewhat conflicting evidence.[18–20] In a large population-based Japanese study, Li and colleagues showed shorter testosterone (TST) in women and later bedtimes.[18] In addition, women older than 50

years had a larger reduction in sleep efficiency with aging, due mainly to increasing durations of nighttime awakening.[18] In contrast, actigraphy data in an elderly population from the Rotterdam study showed women to have longer and less-fragmented sleep than men,[19] which was also supported in a large meta-analysis of data from the Netherlands, United States, and United Kingdom, showing women (>41 years) sleep longer and somewhat more efficiently than men of similar age.[20]

From PG data, several studies have shown lower apnea-hypopnea index (AHI), more partial obstruction, and shorter events in women compared with men.[21–23] In one of the largest studies of polysomnographic features of OSA, O'Connor and colleagues showed[24] that despite similar overall severity of OSA in women and men during rapid eye movement (REM) sleep, women had less severe OSA during NREM sleep.[24] In effect, women therefore seemed to have a higher prevalence of REM-related OSA events.[24] Also, Basoglu and colleagues showed higher REM-AHI in female patients compared with male patients and in addition, lower overall AHI and oxygen desaturation index (ODI), less events in supine position, and at the same time lower mean and lowest oxygen saturation (SaO$_2$).[23] Furthermore, women have shown more respiratory effort–related arousal events and upper airway resistance syndrome.[21,22,24–26] The clinical relevance of these results are still unclear, but it may indicate that women in effect do not have less severe OSA (especially as women seem to have more REM-OSA and hence deeper desaturations) but rather do not in fact fit well with current scoring criteria and hence could be undertreated.

In an attempt to produce normative values for PSG also adjusted for sex and age, Boulos and colleagues compiled data from 169 research studies, comprising 5273 healthy participants and showed female sex was associated with higher REM latency and mean SaO$_2$.[27] Female sex was also associated with lower mean arousal index and lower AHI.[27] In a big data analysis of the dynamics of sleep architecture and effects of individual differences, Yetton and colleagues showed that in addition to sleep architecture being dependent on time of day, total sleep time, and age, sleep architecture also depends on sex.[28] Sex primarily influenced the transition between sleep stages rather than durations of sleep stages, and the investigators state that sex differences in sleep architecture are not due to a reduced tendency to stay in various stages such as SWS but a difficulty in transitioning to them (so-called transition difficulty; ie, going in to for instance SWS).[28]

In addition, interactions between sex and age were apparent, particularly in measure of SWS where women had less deficit in SWS with increasing age. Men on the other hand had less total minutes in SWS as well as reduced proportions of SWS, less probability to transition to SWS, and shorter durations in each SWS epoch.[28] The effect of sex and age on SWS has also been assessed in a data-driven approach by Rosinvil and colleagues aiming to adapt SWS criteria to sex and age. In this data-driven approach, they defined age- and sex-adapted SWS criteria in a cohort of young and older individuals (the so-called learning cohort) based on previous SWS criteria that were adapted to age and sex differences defined in the data-driven process, and then validated the criteria in an independent second cohort (so called testing cohort). In contrast to previous studies showing sex differences, Rosinvil and colleagues showed that when applying the sex- and age-adapted SWS criteria, sex differences vanished, whereas age differences maintained.[29]

The set up for PSG, PG, and actigraphy, respectively, does not specify any differences for women as opposed to men, and scoring criteria are not different between sexes.[11,30] To our knowledge, no studies have assessed whether setup should be different for men and women. However, it has been discussed whether or not signals of PSG are different in men compared with women due to differences in skull characteristics.[31]

Objective Measures of Alertness and Sleepiness

Objective measures of alertness and sleepiness are key tools for diagnosis of excessive somnolence and commonly used in research studies to assess sleepiness. These include the Multiple Sleep Latency Test (MSLT), which measures daytime sleepiness by the propensity to fall asleep during repeated nap opportunities[32,33]; the Maintenance of Wakefulness Test (MWT), which measures ability to stay awake under soporific circumstances, rather than propensity to fall asleep[34]; and the Psychomotor Vigilance task (PVT), which is a reaction-time task testing vigilance[35] and sensitive to sleep deprivation.[36]

Multiple sleep latency test

Studies that include analyses of potential sex differences on the MSLT range from cohorts drawn from in the general population, to various clinical groups. In general, men exhibit shorter sleep latencies,[37–41] and higher prevalence of sleep-onset REM,[41–44] whereas Won and colleagues found shorter sleep onset latency (SOL) in

narcoleptic women.[45] However, several studies find no sex differences in MSLT.[3,46,47]

Maintenance of wakefulness test

As outlined for MSLT, there are reports indicating that men and women might differ in ability to stay awake. Although that is a valid reason to explore potential sex differences also for the MWT, such studies are to a large extent lacking. Sprecher and colleagues[48] investigated sleep restriction and circadian misalignment in 8 women and 12 men, thus not sufficiently powered for analyses of sex differences. However, exploratory analyses did not find differences by sex on MWT.[48] This is in line with Mitler and colleagues who reported no sex differences on MWT in patients with necrolepsy.[49]

Psychomotor vigilance task

Even though PVT is a common tool in research, there are few studies assessing possible differences between women and men in PVT performance.[48,50–53] Blatter and colleagues investigated PVT performance during sleep deprivation and a protocol with multiple naps (lower sleep pressure), showing women in general having slower reaction times compared with men.[51] The investigators speculate that women and men might use different strategies when performing the PVT, because women tended to have fewer instances of premature key presses. This is in line with Batool-Anwar and colleagues in which 61 patients under investigation for OSA performed the PVT.[52] Women tended to have worse performance on the PVT compared with men; however, this result was derived from a subgroup analysis, and the data were not shown in the paper. Sprecher and colleagues[48] also performed exploratory analyses with respect to potential sex differences and found that women performed worse on the PVT; however, only 8 women and 12 men were included in the study. In contrast, Thomann and colleagues did not notice any sex differences on PVT performance in patients with sleep-wake disorders and healthy controls.[53]

Subjective and Semiobjective Sleep-Related Measurements

Sleep diaries

Sleep diaries ask respondents to assess their sleep patterns, (eg, bedtimes, rise times, sleep onset, wake up time) and various other subjective experiences related to sleep quality and/or daytime functioning. Examples of validated sleep diaries include the Pittsburgh Sleep Diary and the Consensus Sleep Diary.[54,55]

Sleep diaries are typically validated against sleep questionnaires, actigraphy, or PSG.[55–57]

Although there are validation studies for some sleep diaries in both nonclinical[57–63] and various clinical samples (eg, insomnia,[64] comorbid insomnia and depression,[14] chronic pain,[65] breast cancer[66]), and most validation studies have included both men and women, gender differences in the measurement properties of sleep diaries are typically not reported. There are some indications, however, that gender might affect the correlation between sleep diary data and other sleep measurements. In a study in community-dwelling elderly comparing sleep diary data, van der Berg and colleagues[62] found that the agreement between total sleep time as assessed by a sleep diary and actigraphy was greater in women than in men and that, in comparison to men, women tended to underestimate their total sleep time in their diaries, whereas men tended to overestimate theirs. However, in another study in older adults, Landry and colleagues[67] reported that gender did not have any marked effect on the association between Consensus Sleep Diary data, Pittsburgh Sleep Quality Index (PSQI), and actigraphy data. Mallinson and colleagues[56] compared the association between sleep diary total sleep time and responses to questions about habitual sleep duration in weekdays and weekends, respectively. They found a larger disagreement between sleep diary and questionnaire data in women than in men, although the difference was small (8 minutes). Miller and colleagues,[68] however, found no significant differences between men and women in a large-scale online study comparing sleep diary data with questions about habitual sleep duration.

Pittsburgh sleep quality index

PSQI was introduced by Buysse and colleagues to assess sleep quality.[69] It results in 7 component scores from 0 to 3, which can be added to a global score ranging from 0 to 21 (with higher scores indicating worse sleep quality and a cutoff score of 5 for good vs poor sleep quality). Most studies regarding psychometric properties of PSQI and gender have either studied gender differences in PSQI scores, in the factorial structure (ie, what items tend to correlate the strongest with each other), or in how PSQI scores are related to other sleep measurements. Regarding PSQI scores, some studies have found no gender differences,[70] whereas others have found gender-based differences[19,71,72] (typically women having higher scores than men, although some have found the opposite[73]) and that aging affects PSQI differently in men and women.[74]

Both 1, 2, and 3 factor solutions have been suggested, as reviewed by Manzar and colleagues.[75]

Morris and colleagues compared the results of separate principal component analyses and parallel analyses of PSQI in men and women, finding different factor loadings in men and women in their 3-factor solution.[76] Although in men overall sleep quality loaded on the same factor as sleep efficiency and sleep duration, in women it loaded with daytime dysfunction and sleep disturbances; this might indicate that men and women mean different things with sleep quality. Li and colleagues, however, found that a 2-factor solution identified using exploratory factor analysis was invariant with regard to gender.[71] Most published factor analyses, however, have not included gender as an explicit covariate or tested for factor invariance across genders.

Aside from grouping items in a questionnaire together into factors, another possible approach to look for gender differences is to focus on subgroups among the respondents, using cluster analysis or latent class analysis. Doing so also allows comparisons of respondent subgroups among men and women. Buysse and colleagues[77] performed a cluster analysis of 187 middle-aged subjects based on their responses on PSQI and Epworth Sleepiness Scale (ESS) and found 4 clusters: low PSQI/low ESS, low PSQI/high ESS, high PSQI/low ESS, and high PSQI/high ESS. Women were significantly more likely than men to end up in the clusters with high PSQI than men. Similar findings were reported by Mondal and colleagues in a clinical sample of patients referred to a sleep clinic.[78] In a gender-specific latent class analysis of a community sample based on their responses to PSQI, Chen and colleagues found that although in men 2 latent classes could be identified (ie, good sleepers and poor sleepers), in women 4 latent classes were defined.[79] Apart from good sleep and poor sleep, there were also latent classes that were termed "inadequate sleep" and "daytime dysfunction," consisting of subjects with PSQI global scores of 7 to 8 with either short sleep duration or significant subjective daytime dysfunction.

Insomnia severity index

Insomnia severity index (ISI) was published in 1993 by Morin, but the first psychometric assessment was published in 2001.[80] ISI scores range from 0 to 28, with higher scores indicating more severe insomnia symptoms. There are several cutoffs: 0 to 7 is considered normal, and 8, 15, and 22 are cutoffs for subthreshold, moderate, and severe insomnia, respectively. Various factor analyses, validations of translated versions, and psychometric evaluations in different patient groups have been published since (eg, primary care patients,[81] patients with cancer,[82] sickle cell anemia patients,[83] military veterans,[84,85] firefighters and rescue workers,[86] and general population[87]). Some studies find higher ISI scores in women,[87,88] but others have failed to find consistent gender differences.[89,90] Factorial invariance across genders have been found reporting solutions with different number of factors[91,92] (ie, the same factor structure is found in men and women, so items that tend to correlate strongly with each other in men also tend to correlate strongly in women and vice versa).

STOP-BANG questionnaire

The STOP-BANG (Snoring, Tiredness, Observed apneas, [high blood] Pressure, Body Mass Index, Age, Neck circumference and Gender) questionnaire[93,94] was developed by Chung and colleagues[95] based on the previously published STOP questionnaire.[94] Its goal is to serve as a risk indicator to classify patients as having a low, moderate, or high risk of OSA.

TOP-BANG scores are by definition sensitive to gender (G stands for "gender"), and men are given a higher score to reflect the higher prevalence of OSA in men.

Several studies and review papers have indicated clinical differences between women and men with OSA,[96–99] with potential relevance to the items in STOP-BANG. Witnessed snoring was a less common presenting symptom in women with OSA than in men in a matched case study.[96] Also, women had lower snoring index than men,[100] but the literature is conflicted as to whether there are any gender differences in snoring intensity.[100,101] Age acts as an effect modifier on the relationship between snoring and gender.[102]

Neither Zhang and colleagues[96] nor Basoglu and colleagues[23] found differences between women and men with OSA regarding daytime sleepiness. Other studies have reported a difference in that men are more likely to report excessive daytime sleepiness, whereas women are more likely to report insomnia or other symptoms that are not explicitly asked for in STOP-BANG.[21,98,103]

Observed apnea is a less common presenting symptom in women than in men,[104] possibly because women with OSA tend to have fewer outright apneas, with more partially obstructive events instead.[98]

There are also indications that the relationship between the risk of having OSA and anthropometric measures (ie, neck circumference and body mass index, in the case of STOP-BANG) is different between men and women. For example, fat distribution is different in men and women,[105] and fat distribution affects the risk of OSA.[106] Adding an item about fat distribution (ie, excess upper body fat) improves the accuracy of STOP-BANG.[107] There is conflicting evidence as to whether neck circumference (which is related to fat distribution) is associated to OSA risk and/or severity in both men and women: Polesel and colleagues,[108] Zhang and colleagues,[96] and Subramanian and colleagues[109] found a correlation between neck circumference and OSA severity in both men and women. Lim and colleagues[110] found neck circumference to be associated to OSA in men but not in women. Onat and colleagues[111] found a correlation between neck circumference and AHI in both men and women, but in a logistic model where presence of OSA was modeled from age, neck circumference, and waist circumference, waist circumference, but not neck circumference, was significantly related to OSA in women.

Age is related to the risk of having OSA, but women tend to get OSA later in life than men,[98] meaning that the Age item might work differently in men and women. There have been studies suggesting alternative scoring criteria or cutoffs for STOP-BANG. Öztürk and colleagues[112] suggested different cutoffs for neck circumference in Turkish men and women, and other studies (not specifically examining STOP-BANG, but neck circumference) have found other cutoffs in other populations.[113,114] Mou and colleagues compared STOP-BANG in patients referred for suspected sleep apnea with regard to its diagnostic accuracy.[115] In summary, they found a low specificity for sleep apnea in men, and with higher AHI, the specificity improved in women but worsened in men. They proposed gender-specific scoring criteria that outperformed traditional scoring. They argue that the Gender item in the traditional STOP-BANG oversimplifies the matter of gender and its effects on OSA likelihood.

Epworth sleepiness scale

ESS was developed by Johns and published in 1991 to assess daytime sleepiness.[116,117] The scale ranges from 0 to 24, with higher scores indicating more daytime sleepiness. There are different findings regarding how ESS scores vary between men and women and to what extent this relationship is affected by age. In a normative sample in the United States,[118] no significant gender differences were found, whereas a German sample found women to report less daytime sleepiness than men.[119] In a meta-regression of factors associated to daytime sleepiness in medical students male gender was not found to be associated with reporting excessive daytime sleepiness.[120]

However, in the Sleep Heart Health Study (SHHS), there was a significant difference with women both having lower mean scores than men and being less likely to score in the excessive daytime sleepiness range.[121] SHHS participants were also asked how often they felt sleepy or unrested, and women were more likely to endorse the "unrested" item, whereas there was no gender difference in the daytime sleepiness item. These findings are also supported by data from the Wisconsin Sleep Cohort.[122] There, 13 items about daytime sleepiness (including all eight items from the ESS) were factor analyzed into 3 factors (perceived sleepiness, sleep propensity in passive situations, and sleep propensity in active situations). The 2 sleep propensity factors mostly consisted of ESS items, and the scores on these factors were higher in men, whereas the perceived sleepiness factor (which consisted of items such as feeling sleepy or needing coffee during the day) was more endorsed in women. However, in a study by Thorarinsdottir and colleagues,[123] where community samples in Sweden and Iceland answered both ESS and the Basic Nordic Sleep Questionnaire (which includes an item about the frequency of feeling sleepy), there was no significant difference in gender distribution among subjects not reporting daytime sleepiness on any of the instruments, ie. people reporting daytime sleepness only on ESS, people reporting it on BNSQ, and people reporting it on both.[123] Differential item functioning with regard to gender was found in one item (item 3, ie, sitting inactive in a public meeting).[124] There is also some evidence that age affects ESS scores differently in men and women. Peak ESS scores in women are reported earlier in life than in men[125,126]: in men, the highest reported level of daytime sleepiness occurs in their seventh decade, whereas it occurs in the third to fifth decade in women. The reasons are not clear.

Chronotype questionnaires

Several questionnaires[127–131] exist to assess chronotype, that is, a subject's inclination to prefer to be asleep or active at different times of the day/night cycle. Although some studies have indicated that women are more likely to express a preference for morningness,[132] others report no gender differences.[133] In the Munich Chronotype Questionnaire, an adjusted score that takes age and gender into account can be applied[134] and is recommended in studies that examine genetics or epidemiology.[135] In a meta-analysis of studies published between 1986 and 2018,[5] the gender differences decreased with increasing age, especially around menopause. There was also an effect of publication year, where the gender difference

was less pronounced in studies published later. The investigators speculate that this might be due to increased gender equality. The choice of instrument used in the studies, however, did not significantly affect the findings. A study by Dutarte and colleagues even suggested a reversal of the gender effect in older subjects (ie, with older men being more morning oriented than older women),[136] but more research is needed in postmenopausal women regarding chronotype.

DISCUSSION

Current evidence show differences in objective measures of sleep, OSA, and sleepiness, including variables from PSG, actigraphy, and PG, as well as MSLT and PVT, between women and men. When discussing the current knowledge, it is important to remember that to date we do not have a consensus on what measure shows "good sleep" and the perception of sleep seems to change with age.[9] Objectively, women show shorter TST, shorter sleep latency, and longer REM sleep latency.[15–20] However, women seem to have less-fragmented sleep, lower arousal index, less NREM stage 1 and 2 sleep, more SWS, and longer bouts of sleep epochs.[27] With increasing age, studies show less delta activity in women compared with men,[27] although there is also contrasting evidence showing women having less deficits in SWS, exhibited by more total minutes in this stage, and less reduced SWS proportions, transition probabilities, and durations as compared with men.[28] As applying age- and sex-adapted SWS criteria to sleep scoring seems to counteract the effect of sex,[29] there is the possibility that age has a stronger effect on sleep variables than sex.[27,29] Measures of sleep apnea also show sex differences, with women exhibiting lower AHI and ODI, more partial occlusion, higher REM-AHI, and less supine AHI.[21–24,27,97,98] Mechanistic explanations for the sleep and sleep apnea differences between sexes have been suggested, such as age, differences in circadian rhythm, and hormones[19] and for OSA, also other factors such as anatomy.[98,137] In women, previous studies have shown increased sleep disruption after menopause[138]; however, studies have also shown the opposite, with postmenopausal women exhibiting increased SWS.[139] Nonetheless, the mechanisms and also the clinical implications of these findings are still not fully elucidated.

Although differences in sleep and sleep apnea have been shown also in meta-analysis,[27,28] there is still a lack of studies in women, and in addition, few studies to date are designed specifically for studying sex or gender differences of sleep variables. This type of study is needed if we are to fully understand sleep differences in women and men. Therefore, future studies need to continue focusing on sex and gender differences and also the interaction with age along with possible effects of sex hormones across the life-span to further explore and determine differences in sleep measures in women compared with men.

Current evidence show some support for sex differences in objective measures of alertness and sleepiness, as there were some indications that results from MSLT can differ between women and men. Specifically, men seem to exhibit shorter sleep latencies and higher prevalence of sleep-onset REM, but there are also studies reporting shorter SOL in women or no sex differences on the MSLT.[3,37–47] Regarding PVT, studies are few and findings mixed. Blatter and colleagues[51] found that women had slower PVT reaction times but also tended to have fewer instances of premature key presses compared with men. It is possible that women and men tend to use different strategies when performing the PVT, even though they are given the same instructions. Considering how common PVT is in research studies, this is an area in urgent need of further investigation.

Clinically, there are today no differences in care guidelines depending on sex or gender but it could be argued that differences in care should depend on sex, as sleep and sleep apnea seem to have different features in women and men. To date, there are also no differences in setup of recording or scoring depending on sex,[11,30] and in addition, it is not elucidated whether or not differences in physical characteristic (for instance skull characteristics[31]) may contribute to differences in signals. Data from Rosinvil and colleagues showed that including sex and also age in their model predictions affected the recorded/analyzed signal (SWS)[29] and that from Yetton and colleagues[28] showed an apparent interaction between sex and age. At least when it comes to the scoring of sleep and sleep-related variables, this raises the important issue of whether or not different scoring criteria should be applied in different groups.

To some extent, the issue of measuring sleep in women is the issue of to what extent gender or sex affects the methods we use to measure sleep, that is, many of the points we raise could also be relevant if the topic had been "measuring sleep in men." It is not simply a question about whether men and women sleep differently or experience their sleep in different ways, although to some extent such differences may matter. If a sleep disorder is more common in one sex, such as OSA in men or insomnia or restless legs in women,[140] a measurement with the same sensitivity and

specificity to detect that disease in men and women, respectively, will have different positive and negative predictive values in men and women.[141] This difference is caused by the fact that the rarer a disease is in a group, the higher is the likelihood that a positive test result will be falsely positive, which in turn leads to a lower positive predictive value in that group.

Regarding questionnaires, gender may affect the psychometric properties in various ways. Many questionnaires are based around the idea of summing scores of several items. In order for such a summed score to be theoretically sound, it is important that the items measure the same thing, or one might be comparing apples with oranges in a sense; this is typically shown using factor analysis, where items are grouped into factors based on their covariance matrix, so items to which the responses are typically strongly correlated are grouped together.[142] It is, however, not necessarily the case that these factors are invariant with regard to gender, that is, items that correlate strongly in men may not correlate in women and vice versa. There are some indications that this is an issue with the PSQI, for example, an instrument for which there are several factor structures published.[71,75,76] Another issue is differential item functioning, where an individual item has different psychometric properties in different groups of respondents (eg, men and women), and this can lead to men and women experiencing the same intensity of a symptom getting different scores on a questionnaire measuring that symptom, thereby creating the illusion of gender differences that are not there or conversely obfuscating gender differences that exist. The ESS, for example, contains items that men and women tend to answer differently. Boyes and colleagues[126] found that men scored higher on items 3 (inactive in a public place), 6 (sitting and talking to someone), 7 (sitting quietly after lunch), and 8 (in a car while stopped for a few minutes in traffic), whereas women scored higher on items 1 (sitting and reading), 4 (as a passenger in a car for an hour without break), and 5 (lying down to rest in the afternoon).

Gender or sex might not only affect how we measure sleep-related phenomena, but it might also act in more complex ways to affect the results of our measurements, especially in clinical settings. In addition to potential physiologic differences between sexes that can affect diagnostic and research outcomes, it is possible that women and men can differ in how they perceive and report their symptoms, likelihood to seek medical care, and filling in questionnaires and strategies used on cognitive tests.[45,51,56,68,143,144] These factors could in turn be affected by norms, differences in expectations between women and men, life situation, and personality. The first assessment of a patient is typically not through a formal measurement but a clinical assessment based on history taking and a physical examination. If clinicians have preconceptions that make them less likely to suspect, for instance OSA in a woman, not for actual clinical reasons but the patient might not fit into the OSA stereotype of a middle-aged, overweight, sleepy man, they may be less likely to refer the patient to further examination.[145–147] Taking narcolepsy as an additional example, both men and women can be affected, but there is a substantial sex difference in time from symptom onset to diagnosis.[148] Won and colleagues mark that even though men and women present with similar symptoms of narcolepsy, 85% of men were likely to be diagnosed within 16 years, whereas 85% of women were likely to be diagnosed within 28 years from symptoms onset[45]; this is concerning and might influence disease progression and quality of life. In order to take preventive measures, it is important to consider possible causes behind this pattern, which also brings us to the core of this review: are there sex differences in sleep-related functions, and are our diagnostic and research tools sufficiently developed to take these sex and gender differences into account?

Most methods and instruments in this review have not been substantially tested for sex or gender differences, and only few studies had the primary aim to investigate sex differences; this is problematic, as potential sex differences might have been missed, thus risking that standard values are misleading, diagnoses missed or delayed, and results from scientific studies could be distorted. In combination with referral selection bias, affected by the clinician's preconceptions and knowledge, methodological tools not sensitive enough to detect potential sex or gender differences could possibly be contributing to delay diagnoses in women for certain sleep disorders.

FUTURE DIRECTIONS

Although differences between women and men have been shown for subjective and objective sleep measures, there is still a lack of studies in women, and in addition, few studies have been aimed and designed specifically for looking at sex differences in sleep measurements. Therefore, it is of importance that future studies have a greater focus on potential sex differences.

In addition to what we have covered in this review, there is a great need for future studies to further examine the effect of the menstrual cycle and hormonal contraceptives on sleep and sleep-related functions and related methods.[149] Today, menstrual cycle status and hormonal contraceptive use is taken into account differently between studies but most often not at all.

Not only the measurements themselves but also how we talk and write about differences between women and men are important. As scientists and health professionals, we need to be aware of the importance of phrasing for setting standards. Do we refer to men's symptoms as typical, whereas women's symptoms are atypical because they are less studied?

It is also common that the terms "gender" and "sex" are used as equivalents, and there seems to be some confusion regarding when the one or the other are more appropriate to use; this is outside of the scope of this review but something we suggest that journals should have guidelines for and writers and reviewers be aware of. To conclude, words matter.

SUMMARY

In sum, although it is likely that there are differences in sleep between women and men, which has also been shown in large meta-analyses, few studies to date are specifically designed to study sex or gender differences of sleep variables, and measurements are not sufficiently validated with respect to sex differences. These types of studies are needed if we are to fully understand sleep and sleep disorders in women and men. Future studies need to focus on sex and gender differences and the interaction with age, along with possible effects of sex hormones across the life-span. We urge researchers, policy makers, and clinicians to reflect on the consequences of not studying sex differences and to take steps to increase equality in research, method development, guidelines, and health care.

CLINICS CARE POINTS

- Both objective and subjective measures of sleep and sleep-related variables show differences between women and men in some aspects.

- Most methods and instruments assessing sleep have not been substantially tested for sex or gender differences, and only few studies have had the primary aim to investigate sex differences.

- There are to date no guidelines as to whether or not scoring (or set up) should be performed differently in women and men, and studies to assess whether different approaches should be applied are needed.
- Future studies need to be specifically designed to study sex or gender differences of sleep variables and focus on sex and gender differences and the interaction with age, along with possible effects of sex hormones across the life-span.

DISCLOSURE

J. Theorell-Haglöw and M. Ulander have nothing to disclose. F. Rångtell is the founder of Slumra of Sweden in which she gives payed lectures and scientific consultancy within the sleep field. F. Rångtell has acted as scientific advisor or content writer for several organizations and sleep-related companies, including Sleep Cycle and The Nap lab. None of FR's collaborations had any insight into or influence on the work related to this article.

REFERENCES

1. Zhang B, Wing YK. Sex differences in insomnia: a meta-analysis. Sleep 2006;29(1):85–93.
2. Bixler EO, Papaliaga MN, Vgontzas AN, et al. Women sleep objectively better than men and the sleep of young women is more resilient to external stressors: effects of age and menopause. J Sleep Res 2009;18(2):221–8.
3. Roehrs T, Kapke A, Roth T, et al. Sex differences in the polysomnographic sleep of young adults: a community-based study. Sleep Med 2006;7(1):49–53.
4. Walsleben JA, Kapur VK, Newman AB, et al. Sleep and reported daytime sleepiness in normal subjects: the Sleep Heart Health Study. Sleep 2004;27(2):293–8.
5. Randler C, Engelke J. Gender differences in chronotype diminish with age: a meta-analysis based on morningness/chronotype questionnaires. Chronobiol Int 2019;36(7):888–905.
6. Calhoun SL, Fernandez-Mendoza J, Vgontzas AN, et al. Prevalence of insomnia symptoms in a general population sample of young children and pre-adolescents: gender effects. Sleep Med 2014;15(1):91–5.
7. Krishnan V, Collop NA. Gender differences in sleep disorders. Curr Opin Pulm Med 2006;12(6):383–9.
8. Knutson KL. The association between pubertal status and sleep duration and quality among a nationally representative sample of U. S. adolescents. Am J Hum Biol 2005;17(4):418–24.
9. Akerstedt T, Schwarz J, Gruber G, et al. The relation between polysomnography and subjective sleep and its dependence on age - poor sleep may become good sleep. J Sleep Res 2016;25(5):565–70.
10. Rechtschaffen A, Kales A. A manual of standardized terminology, techniques, and scoring system for sleep stages in human subjects. Washington (D.C.): U.S National Public Health Service, U.S. Government Printing Office; 1968.
11. Berry RB, Brooks R, Gamaldo C, et al. AASM scoring manual updates for 2017 (version 2.4). J Clin Sleep Med 2017;13(5):665–6.
12. Ancoli-Israel S, Cole R, Alessi C, et al. The role of actigraphy in the study of sleep and circadian rhythms. Sleep 2003;26(3):342–92.
13. Paquet J, Kawinska A, Carrier J. Wake detection capacity of actigraphy during sleep. Sleep 2007;30(10):1362–9.
14. McCall C, McCall WV. Comparison of actigraphy with polysomnography and sleep logs in depressed insomniacs. J Sleep Res 2012;21(1):122–7.
15. Ohayon MM, Reynolds CF 3rd, Dauvilliers Y. Excessive sleep duration and quality of life. Ann Neurol 2013;73(6):785–94.
16. Redline S, Kirchner HL, Quan SF, et al. The effects of age, sex, ethnicity, and sleep-disordered breathing on sleep architecture. Arch Intern Med 2004;164(4):406–18.
17. Latta F, Leproult R, Tasali E, et al. Sex differences in delta and alpha EEG activities in healthy older adults. Sleep 2005;28(12):1525–34.
18. Li L, Nakamura T, Hayano J, et al. Age and gender differences in objective sleep properties using large-scale body acceleration data in a Japanese population. Sci Rep 2021;11(1):9970.
19. van den Berg JF, Miedema HM, Tulen JH, et al. Sex differences in subjective and actigraphic sleep measures: a population-based study of elderly persons. Sleep 2009;32(10):1367–75.
20. Kocevska D, Lysen TS, Dotinga A, et al. Sleep characteristics across the lifespan in 1.1 million people from The Netherlands, United Kingdom and United States: a systematic review and meta-analysis. Nat Hum Behav 2021;5(1):113–22.
21. Valipour A, Lothaller H, Rauscher H, et al. Gender-related differences in symptoms of patients with suspected breathing disorders in sleep: a clinical population study using the sleep disorders questionnaire. Sleep 2007;30(3):312–9.
22. Ye L, Pien GW, Weaver TE. Gender differences in the clinical manifestation of obstructive sleep apnea. Sleep Med 2009;10(10):1075–84.
23. Basoglu OK, Tasbakan MS. Gender differences in clinical and polysomnographic features of obstructive sleep apnea: a clinical study of 2827 patients. Sleep Breath 2018;22(1):241–9.

24. O'Connor C, Thornley KS, Hanly PJ. Gender differences in the polysomnographic features of obstructive sleep apnea. Am J Respir Crit Care Med 2000;161(5):1465–72.

25. Gabbay IE, Lavie P. Age- and gender-related characteristics of obstructive sleep apnea. Sleep Breath 2012;16(2):453–60.

26. Koo BB, Dostal J, Ioachimescu O, et al. The effects of gender and age on REM-related sleep-disordered breathing. Sleep Breath 2008;12(3):259–64.

27. Boulos MI, Jairam T, Kendzerska T, et al. Normal polysomnography parameters in healthy adults: a systematic review and meta-analysis. Lancet Respir Med 2019;7(6):533–43.

28. Yetton BD, McDevitt EA, Cellini N, et al. Quantifying sleep architecture dynamics and individual differences using big data and Bayesian networks. PLoS One 2018;13(4):e0194604.

29. Rosinvil T, Bouvier J, Dube J, et al. Are age and sex effects on sleep slow waves only a matter of electroencephalogram amplitude? Sleep 2021;44(3).

30. Fekedulegn D, Andrew ME, Shi M, et al. Actigraphy-based assessment of sleep parameters. Ann Work Expo Health 2020;64(4):350–67.

31. Dijk DJ, Beersma DG, Bloem GM. Sex differences in the sleep EEG of young adults: visual scoring and spectral analysis. Sleep 1989;12(6):500–7.

32. Carskadon MA, Dement WC. Effects of total sleep loss on sleep tendency. Percept Mot Skills 1979; 48(2):495–506.

33. Carskadon MA, Dement WC, Mitler MM, et al. Guidelines for the multiple sleep latency test (MSLT): a standard measure of sleepiness. Sleep 1986;9(4):519–24.

34. Doghramji K, Mitler MM, Sangal RB, et al. A normative study of the maintenance of wakefulness test (MWT). Electroencephalogr Clin Neurophysiol 1997;103(5):554–62.

35. Van Dongen HP, Maislin G, Mullington JM, et al. The cumulative cost of additional wakefulness: dose-response effects on neurobehavioral functions and sleep physiology from chronic sleep restriction and total sleep deprivation. Sleep 2003;26(2):117–26.

36. Dinges DF, Powell JW. Microcomputer analyses of performance on a portable, simple visual rt task during sustained operations. Behav Res Meth Instr 1985;17(6):652–5.

37. Geisler P, Tracik F, Cronlein T, et al. The influence of age and sex on sleep latency in the MSLT-30–a normative study. Sleep 2006;29(5):687–92.

38. Punjabi NM, Bandeen-Roche K, Young T. Predictors of objective sleep tendency in the general population. Sleep 2003;26(6):678–83.

39. Kainulainen S, Toyras J, Oksenberg A, et al. Severity of desaturations reflects OSA-related daytime sleepiness better than AHI. J Clin Sleep Med 2019;15(8):1135–42.

40. Ali M, Auger RR, Slocumb NL, et al. Idiopathic hypersomnia: clinical features and response to treatment. J Clin Sleep Med 2009;5(6):562–8.

41. Goldbart A, Peppard P, Finn L, et al. Narcolepsy and predictors of positive MSLTs in the Wisconsin sleep cohort. Sleep 2014;37(6):1043–51.

42. Mignot E, Lin L, Finn L, et al. Correlates of sleep-onset REM periods during the multiple sleep latency test in community adults. Brain 2006;129(Pt 6):1609–23.

43. Cairns A, Trotti LM, Bogan R. Demographic and nap-related variance of the MSLT: results from 2,498 suspected hypersomnia patients: clinical MSLT variance. Sleep Med 2019;55:115–23.

44. Chervin RD, Aldrich MS. Sleep onset REM periods during multiple sleep latency tests in patients evaluated for sleep apnea. Am J Respir Crit Care Med 2000;161(2 Pt 1):426–31.

45. Won C, Mahmoudi M, Qin L, et al. The impact of gender on timeliness of narcolepsy diagnosis. J Clin Sleep Med 2014;10(1):89–95.

46. Kronholm E, Hyyppa MT, Alanen E, et al. What does the multiple sleep latency test measure in a community sample? Sleep 1995;18(10):827–35.

47. Briones B, Adams N, Strauss M, et al. Relationship between sleepiness and general health status. Sleep 1996;19(7):583–8.

48. Sprecher KE, Ritchie HK, Burke TM, et al. Trait-like vulnerability of higher-order cognition and ability to maintain wakefulness during combined sleep restriction and circadian misalignment. Sleep 2019; 42(8).

49. Mitler MM, Walsleben J, Sangal RB, et al. Sleep latency on the maintenance of wakefulness test (MWT) for 530 patients with narcolepsy while free of psychoactive drugs. Electroencephalogr Clin Neurophysiol 1998;107(1):33–8.

50. Vidafar P, Gooley JJ, Burns AC, et al. Increased vulnerability to attentional failure during acute sleep deprivation in women depends on menstrual phase. Sleep 2018;41(8).

51. Blatter K, Graw P, Munch M, et al. Gender and age differences in psychomotor vigilance performance under differential sleep pressure conditions. Behav Brain Res 2006;168(2):312–7.

52. Batool-Anwar S, Kales SN, Patel SR, et al. Obstructive sleep apnea and psychomotor vigilance task performance. Nat Sci Sleep 2014;6:65–71.

53. Thomann J, Baumann CR, Landolt HP, et al. Psychomotor vigilance task demonstrates impaired vigilance in disorders with excessive daytime sleepiness. J Clin Sleep Med 2014;10(9):1019–24.

54. Carney CE, Buysse DJ, Ancoli-Israel S, et al. The consensus sleep diary: standardizing prospective sleep self-monitoring. Sleep 2012;35(2):287–302.

55. Monk TH, Reynolds CF, Kupfer DJ, et al. The Pittsburgh sleep diary. J Sleep Res 1994;3(2):111–20.

56. Mallinson DC, Kamenetsky ME, Hagen EW, et al. Subjective sleep measurement: comparing sleep diary to questionnaire. Nat Sci Sleep 2019;11:197–206.

57. Dietch JR, Taylor DJ. Evaluation of the Consensus Sleep Diary in a community sample: comparison with single-channel EEG, actigraphy, and retrospective questionnaire. J Clin Sleep Med 2021;17(7):1389–99.

58. Aili K, Astrom-Paulsson S, Stoetzer U, et al. Reliability of actigraphy and subjective sleep measurements in adults: the design of sleep assessments. J Clin Sleep Med 2017;13(1):39–47.

59. Campanini MZ, Lopez-Garcia E, Rodriguez-Artalejo F, et al. Agreement between sleep diary and actigraphy in a highly educated Brazilian population. Sleep Med 2017;35:27–34.

60. Liu J, Wong WT, Zwetsloot IM, et al. Preliminary agreement on tracking sleep between a wrist-worn device fitbit alta and consensus sleep diary. Telemed J E Health 2019;25(12):1189–97.

61. Doroudgar S, Talwar M, Burrowes S, et al. Use of actigraphy and sleep diaries to assess sleep and academic performance in pharmacy students. Curr Pharm Teach Learn 2021;13(1):57–62.

62. Van Den Berg JF, Van Rooij FJ, Vos H, et al. Disagreement between subjective and actigraphic measures of sleep duration in a population-based study of elderly persons. J Sleep Res 2008;17(3):295–302.

63. Dietch JR, Sethi K, Slavish DC, et al. Validity of two retrospective questionnaire versions of the Consensus Sleep Diary: the whole week and split week Self-Assessment of Sleep Surveys. Sleep Med 2019;63:127–36.

64. Maich KHG, Lachowski AM, Carney CE. Psychometric properties of the consensus sleep diary in those with insomnia disorder. Behav Sleep Med 2018;16(2):117–34.

65. Haythornthwaite JA, Hegel MT, Kerns RD. Development of a sleep diary for chronic pain patients. J Pain Symptom Manage 1991;6(2):65–72.

66. Moore CM, Schmiege SJ, Matthews EE. Actigraphy and sleep diary measurements in breast cancer survivors: discrepancy in selected sleep parameters. Behav Sleep Med 2015;13(6):472–90.

67. Landry GJ, Best JR, Liu-Ambrose T. Measuring sleep quality in older adults: a comparison using subjective and objective methods. Front Aging Neurosci 2015;7:166.

68. Miller CB, Gordon CJ, Toubia L, et al. Agreement between simple questions about sleep duration and sleep diaries in a large online survey. Sleep Health 2015;1(2):133–7.

69. Buysse DJ, Reynolds CF 3rd, Monk TH, et al. The Pittsburgh Sleep Quality Index: a new instrument for psychiatric practice and research. Psychiatry Res 1989;28(2):193–213.

70. Buysse DJ, Reynolds CF 3rd, Monk TH, et al. Quantification of subjective sleep quality in healthy elderly men and women using the Pittsburgh Sleep Quality Index (PSQI). Sleep 1991;14(4):331–8.

71. Li L, Sheehan CM, Thompson MS. Measurement invariance and sleep quality differences between men and women in the pittsburgh sleep quality index. J Clin Sleep Med 2019;15(12):1769–76.

72. Lee SY, Ju YJ, Lee JE, et al. Factors associated with poor sleep quality in the Korean general population: providing information from the Korean version of the Pittsburgh Sleep Quality Index. J Affect Disord 2020;271:49–58.

73. Becker SP, Jarrett MA, Luebbe AM, et al. Sleep in a large, multi-university sample of college students: sleep problem prevalence, sex differences, and mental health correlates. Sleep Health 2018;4(2):174–81.

74. Kim HJ, Kim REY, Kim S, et al. Sex differences in deterioration of sleep properties associated with aging: a 12-year longitudinal cohort study. J Clin Sleep Med 2021;17(5):964–72.

75. Manzar MD, BaHammam AS, Hameed UA, et al. Dimensionality of the Pittsburgh Sleep Quality Index: a systematic review. Health Qual Life Outcomes 2018;16(1):89.

76. Morris JL, Rohay J, Chasens ER. Sex differences in the psychometric properties of the Pittsburgh Sleep Quality Index. J Womens Health (Larchmt) 2018;27(3):278–82.

77. Buysse DJ, Hall ML, Strollo PJ, et al. Relationships between the Pittsburgh Sleep Quality Index (PSQI), Epworth Sleepiness Scale (ESS), and clinical/polysomnographic measures in a community sample. J Clin Sleep Med 2008;4(6):563–71.

78. Mondal P, Gjevre JA, Taylor-Gjevre RM, et al. Relationship between the Pittsburgh Sleep Quality Index and the Epworth Sleepiness Scale in a sleep laboratory referral population. Nat Sci Sleep 2013;5:15–21.

79. Chen X, Fang Y, Liu X, et al. Gender differences in latent classes of sleep quality in community-dwelling adults based on the Pittsburgh sleep quality index. Psychol Health Med 2019;24(8):901–10.

80. Bastien CH, Vallieres A, Morin CM. Validation of the Insomnia Severity Index as an outcome measure for insomnia research. Sleep Med 2001;2(4):297–307.

81. Gagnon C, Belanger L, Ivers H, et al. Validation of the Insomnia Severity Index in primary care. J Am Board Fam Med 2013;26(6):701–10.

82. Savard MH, Savard J, Simard S, Ivers H. Empirical validation of the Insomnia Severity Index in cancer patients. Psychooncology 2005;14(6):429–41.

83. Moscou-Jackson G, Allen J, Smith MT, et al. Psychometric validation of the Insomnia Severity Index in adults with sickle cell disease. J Health Care Poor Underserved 2016;27(1):209–18.

84. Kaufmann CN, Orff HJ, Moore RC, et al. Psychometric characteristics of the Insomnia Severity Index in veterans with history of traumatic brain injury. Behav Sleep Med 2019;17(1):12–8.

85. Wallace DM, Wohlgemuth WK. Predictors of Insomnia Severity Index Profiles in United States veterans with obstructive sleep apnea. J Clin Sleep Med 2019;15(12):1827–37.

86. Jeong HS, Jeon Y, Ma J, et al. Validation of the athens insomnia Scale for screening insomnia in South Korean firefighters and rescue workers. Qual Life Res 2015;24(10):2391–5.

87. Filosa J, Omland PM, Langsrud K, et al. Validation of insomnia questionnaires in the general population: the Nord-Trondelag Health Study (HUNT). J Sleep Res 2021;30(1):e13222.

88. La YK, Choi YH, Chu MK, et al. Gender differences influence over insomnia in Korean population: a cross-sectional study. PLoS One 2020;15(1): e0227190.

89. Gerber M, Lang C, Lemola S, et al. Validation of the German version of the insomnia severity index in adolescents, young adults and adult workers: results from three cross-sectional studies. BMC Psychiatry 2016;16:174.

90. Dieperink KB, Elnegaard CM, Winther B, et al. Preliminary validation of the insomnia severity index in Danish outpatients with a medical condition. J Patient Rep Outcomes 2020;4(1):18.

91. Dragioti E, Wiklund T, Alfoldi P, et al. The Swedish version of the Insomnia Severity Index: factor structure analysis and psychometric properties in chronic pain patients. Scand J Pain 2015;9(1):22–7.

92. Albougami A, Manzar MD. Insomnia severity index: a psychometric investigation among Saudi nurses. Sleep Breath 2019;23(3):987–96.

93. Farney RJ, Walker BS, Farney RM, et al. The STOP-Bang equivalent model and prediction of severity of obstructive sleep apnea: relation to polysomnographic measurements of the apnea/hypopnea index. J Clin Sleep Med 2011;7(5):459–465B.

94. Chung F, Yegneswaran B, Liao P, et al. STOP questionnaire: a tool to screen patients for obstructive sleep apnea. Anesthesiology 2008;108(5):812–21.

95. Chung F, Abdullah HR, Liao P. STOP-bang questionnaire: a practical approach to screen for obstructive sleep apnea. Chest 2016;149(3):631–8.

96. Zhang Z, Cheng J, Yang W, et al. Gender differences in clinical manifestations and polysomnographic findings in Chinese patients with obstructive sleep apnea. Sleep Breath 2020;24(3):1019–26.

97. Valipour A. Gender-related differences in the obstructive sleep apnea syndrome. Pneumologie 2012;66(10):584–8.

98. Bonsignore MR, Saaresranta T, Riha RL. Sex differences in obstructive sleep apnoea. Eur Respir Rev 2019;28(154).

99. Wimms A, Woehrle H, Ketheeswaran S, et al. Obstructive sleep apnea in women: specific issues and interventions. Biomed Res Int 2016;2016: 1764837.

100. Levartovsky A, Dafna E, Zigel Y, et al. Breathing and snoring sound characteristics during sleep in adults. J Clin Sleep Med 2016;12(3):375–84.

101. Pevernagie D, Aarts RM, De Meyer M. The acoustics of snoring. Sleep Med Rev 2010;14(2):131–44.

102. Chan CH, Wong BM, Tang JL, et al. Gender difference in snoring and how it changes with age: systematic review and meta-regression. Sleep Breath 2012;16(4):977–86.

103. Sforza E, Chouchou F, Collet P, et al. Sex differences in obstructive sleep apnoea in an elderly French population. Eur Respir J 2011;37(5):1137–43.

104. Quintana-Gallego E, Carmona-Bernal C, Capote F, et al. Gender differences in obstructive sleep apnea syndrome: a clinical study of 1166 patients. Respir Med 2004;98(10):984–9.

105. Palmer BF, Clegg DJ. The sexual dimorphism of obesity. Mol Cell Endocrinol 2015;402:113–9.

106. Martinez-Rivera C, Abad J, Fiz JA, et al. Usefulness of truncal obesity indices as predictive factors for obstructive sleep apnea syndrome. Obesity (Silver Spring) 2008;16(1):113–8.

107. Sangkum L, Klair I, Limsuwat C, et al. Incorporating body-type (apple vs. pear) in STOP-BANG questionnaire improves its validity to detect OSA. J Clin Anesth 2017;41:126–31.

108. Polesel DN, Nozoe KT, Tufik SB, et al. Gender differences in the application of anthropometric measures for evaluation of obstructive sleep apnea. Sleep Sci 2019;12(1):2–9.

109. Subramanian S, Jayaraman G, Majid H, et al. Influence of gender and anthropometric measures on severity of obstructive sleep apnea. Sleep Breath 2012;16(4):1091–5.

110. Lim YH, Choi J, Kim KR, et al. Sex-specific characteristics of anthropometry in patients with obstructive sleep apnea: neck circumference and waist-hip ratio. Ann Otol Rhinol Laryngol 2014;123(7):517–23.

111. Onat A, Hergenc G, Yuksel H, et al. Neck circumference as a measure of central obesity: associations with metabolic syndrome and obstructive sleep apnea syndrome beyond waist circumference. Clin Nutr 2009;28(1):46–51.

112. Ozturk NAA, Dilektasli AG, Cetinoglu ED, et al. Diagnostic accuracy of a modified STOP-BANG questionnaire with national anthropometric obesity indexes. Turk Thorac J 2019;20(2):103–7.

113. Ruiz AJ, Rondon Sepulveda MA, Franco OH, et al. The associations between sleep disorders and anthropometric measures in adults from three Colombian cities at different altitudes. Maturitas 2016;94:1–10.

114. Simpson L, Mukherjee S, Cooper MN, et al. Sex differences in the association of regional fat distribution with the severity of obstructive sleep apnea. Sleep 2010;33(4):467–74.

115. Mou J, Pflugeisen BM, Crick BA, et al. The discriminative power of STOP-Bang as a screening tool for suspected obstructive sleep apnea in clinically referred patients: considering gender differences. Sleep Breath 2019;23(1):65–75.

116. Johns MW. A new method for measuring daytime sleepiness: the Epworth sleepiness scale. Sleep 1991;14(6):540–5.

117. Johns MW. Sleep propensity varies with behaviour and the situation in which it is measured: the concept of somnificity. J Sleep Res 2002;11(1):61–7.

118. Sanford SD, Lichstein KL, Durrence HH, et al. The influence of age, gender, ethnicity, and insomnia on Epworth sleepiness scores: a normative US population. Sleep Med 2006;7(4):319–26.

119. Sander C, Hegerl U, Wirkner K, et al. Normative values of the Epworth Sleepiness Scale (ESS), derived from a large German sample. Sleep Breath 2016;20(4):1337–45.

120. Jahrami H, Alshomili H, Almannai N, et al. Predictors of excessive daytime sleepiness in medical students: a meta-regression. Clocks Sleep 2019;1(2):209–19.

121. Baldwin CM, Kapur VK, Holberg CJ, et al. Associations between gender and measures of daytime somnolence in the Sleep Heart Health Study. Sleep 2004;27(2):305–11.

122. Kim H, Young T. Subjective daytime sleepiness: dimensions and correlates in the general population. Sleep 2005;28(5):625–34.

123. Thorarinsdottir EH, Bjornsdottir E, Benediktsdottir B, et al. Definition of excessive daytime sleepiness in the general population: feeling sleepy relates better to sleep-related symptoms and quality of life than the Epworth Sleepiness Scale score. Results from an epidemiological study. J Sleep Res 2019;28(6):e12852.

124. Ulander M, Arestedt K, Svanborg E, et al. The fairness of the Epworth Sleepiness Scale: two approaches to differential item functioning. Sleep Breath 2013;17(1):157–65.

125. Drakatos P, Ghiassi R, Jarrold I, et al. The use of an online pictorial Epworth Sleepiness Scale in the assessment of age and gender specific differences in excessive daytime sleepiness. J Thorac Dis 2015;7(5):897–902.

126. Boyes J, Drakatos P, Jarrold I, et al. The use of an online Epworth Sleepiness Scale to assess excessive daytime sleepiness. Sleep Breath 2017;21(2):333–40.

127. Smith CS, Reilly C, Midkiff K. Evaluation of three circadian rhythm questionnaires with suggestions

128. Horne JA, Ostberg O. A self-assessment questionnaire to determine morningness-eveningness in human circadian rhythms. Int J Chronobiol 1976;4(2):97–110.

129. Roenneberg T, Hut R, Daan S, et al. Entrainment concepts revisited. J Biol Rhythms 2010;25(5):329–39.

130. Roenneberg T, Wirz-Justice A, Merrow M. Life between clocks: daily temporal patterns of human chronotypes. J Biol Rhythms 2003;18(1):80–90.

131. Smith CS, Folkard S, Schmieder RA, et al. Investigation of morning-evening orientation in six countries using the preferences scale. Pers Individ Dif 2002;32(6):949–68.

132. Adan A, Natale V. Gender differences in morningness-eveningness preference. Chronobiol Int 2002;19(4):709–20.

133. Caci H, Deschaux O, Adan A, et al. Comparing three morningness scales: age and gender effects, structure and cut-off criteria. Sleep Med 2009;10(2):240–5.

134. Roenneberg T, Kumar CJ, Merrow M. The human circadian clock entrains to sun time. Curr Biol 2007;17(2):R44–5.

135. Roenneberg T, Kuehnle T, Juda M, et al. Epidemiology of the human circadian clock. Sleep Med Rev 2007;11(6):429–38.

136. Duarte LL, Menna-Barreto L, Miguel MA, et al. Chronotype ontogeny related to gender. Braz J Med Biol Res 2014;47(4):316–20.

137. Lindberg E, Bonsignore MR, Polo-Kantola P. Role of menopause and hormone replacement therapy in sleep-disordered breathing. Sleep Med Rev 2020;49:101225.

138. Baker FC, Willoughby AR, Sassoon SA, et al. Insomnia in women approaching menopause: beyond perception. Psychoneuroendocrinology 2015;60:96–104.

139. Young T, Rabago D, Zgierska A, et al. Objective and subjective sleep quality in premenopausal, perimenopausal, and postmenopausal women in the Wisconsin Sleep Cohort Study. Sleep 2003;26(6):667–72.

140. Theorell-Haglow J, Miller CB, Bartlett DJ, et al. Gender differences in obstructive sleep apnoea, insomnia and restless legs syndrome in adults - what do we know? A clinical update. Sleep Med Rev 2018;38:28–38.

141. Brenner H, Gefeller O. Variation of sensitivity, specificity, likelihood ratios and predictive values with disease prevalence. Stat Med 1997;16(9):981–91.

142. Streiner DL, Norman GR. Health measurement scales : a practical guide to their development and use. 4th edition. Oxford (NY): Oxford University Press; 2008.

143. Hohn A, Gampe J, Lindahl-Jacobsen R, et al. Do men avoid seeking medical advice? A register-

based analysis of gender-specific changes in primary healthcare use after first hospitalisation at ages 60+ in Denmark. J Epidemiol Community Health 2020;74(7):573–9.

144. Mallampalli MP, Carter CL. Exploring sex and gender differences in sleep health: a Society for Women's Health Research Report. J Womens Health (Larchmt) 2014;23(7):553–62.

145. Larsson LG, Lindberg A, Franklin KA, et al. Gender differences in symptoms related to sleep apnea in a general population and in relation to referral to sleep clinic. Chest 2003;124(1):204–11.

146. Morris JL, Chasens ER, Brush LD. Gender as a principle of the organization of clinical sleep research. Nurs Outlook 2020;68(6):763–8.

147. Lindberg E, Benediktsdottir B, Franklin KA, et al. Women with symptoms of sleep-disordered breathing are less likely to be diagnosed and treated for sleep apnea than men. Sleep Med 2017;35:17–22.

148. Luca G, Haba-Rubio J, Dauvilliers Y, et al. Clinical, polysomnographic and genome-wide association analyses of narcolepsy with cataplexy: a European Narcolepsy Network study. J Sleep Res 2013; 22(5):482–95.

149. Lord C, Sekerovic Z, Carrier J. Sleep regulation and sex hormones exposure in men and women across adulthood. Pathol Biol (Paris) 2014;62(5): 302–10.

Sleep Measurement in Children—Are We on the Right Track?

Barbara Gnidovec Stražišar, MD, PhD[a,b,c],*

KEYWORDS

- Sleep measurement • Children • Subjective data • Objective data • Autonomic signal assessment
- Sleep diaries • Sleep questionnaires • Actigraphy • Home sleep apnea testing
- In-lab polysomnography • Biomarkers

KEY POINTS

- Sleep disorders in children are prevelent and can have possible serious consequences for their health, development and academic performance.
- Detection of sleep and sleep disorders in children therefore requires valid sleep measures.
- In-laboratory full-night polysomnography is the gold standard for the evaluation of sleep and sleep disorders in children.
- Many other subjective and objective methods are available to evaluate various aspects of sleep in childhood, each with their strenghts and limitation.
- A combination of different instruments along with thorough clinical interview and physical examination provides best insight in child's sleep and its disorders.

INTRODUCTION

Sleep is one of the primary activities of the brain during early development. It is essential for development, maturation, and health of a growing child. Sleep also plays a critical role in learning, attention, memory, and emotional regulation.[1] Thus, it is not surprising that sleep represents more than three-quarters of the life of a newborn, around half of the life of an infant, toddler, and/or a young child, and still at least 8 hours of the life of a teenager.

Pediatric sleep disorders are very frequent and in light of their prevalence and possible serious consequences, it is essential to accurately measure sleep and sleep quality in children. There are numerous methods to measure sleep (for recent review see Arnardottir and colleagues[2]

2021). However, as in many other instances, it is true that children are not just small adults. Besides decreasing need for normal sleep duration in children there are also significant developmental changes in sleep architecture and sleep patterns.[3] Therefore, one must be very careful in making child modification of adult tools or their application beyond the intended age range. Different methods are used to evaluate various aspects of sleep in childhood; some methods are subjective or self-reported, whereas others are objective.

SUBJECTIVE METHODS
Sleep Diaries and Sleep logs

Sleep diaries and sleep logs are important tools for tracking sleep, monitoring sleep habits, and documenting sleep problem. They are widely used in

[a] Pediatric Department, Centre for Pediatric Sleep Disorders, General Hospital Celje, Oblakova ulica 5, Celje 3000, Slovenia; [b] College of Nursing in Celje, Celje, Slovenia; [c] Medical Faculty, University of Maribor, Maribor, Slovenia
* Pediatric Department, Centre for Pediatric Sleep Disorders, General Hospital Celje, Oblakova ulica 5, Celje 3000, Slovenia.
E-mail address: Barbara.gnidovec-strazisar@sb-celje.si

Sleep Med Clin 16 (2021) 649–660
https://doi.org/10.1016/j.jsmc.2021.08.004

sleep research and clinical practice and are considered the gold standard for subjective sleep assessment.[4] Sleep diary represents a daily record of important sleep-related information that commonly include details about bedtime and/or time of lights-out, wake-up time, sleep latency, the number and duration of sleep interruptions, the number and duration of daytime naps, and sometimes also perceived sleep quality. There are numerous different types of sleep diaries and many contain one short section to complete in the morning and another in the evening. Depending on age, they can be completed by the child himself or by his caregiver. The term "sleep diary" is used interchangeably with sleep log, although some consider a sleep diary to be more detailed than a sleep log.[5]

For accurate estimates of typical sleep from daily diaries it is important to take into account intraindividual night-to-night variability in sleep patterns resulting from situational and other influences; this can be reduced by aggregation of multiple nights of sleep estimates.[6] The number of sleep diary nights needed for reliable sleep patterns estimate depends on different factors, including the aspect of sleep assessed (ie, sleep onset latency, total sleep time), the period of sleep aggregated (ie, school night sleep vs weekend sleep), and the sample population (age, healthy individuals vs those with clinical sleep disorders).[6] However, probably the most decisive of all is individual sleep stability, and especially adolescence is characterized by lower individual sleep stability.[7] Short and colleagues[8] therefore recommended that at least 5 weekday nights of sleep diary entries be made when studying adolescent bedtimes, sleep latency, and sleep duration. However, in everyday clinical practice sleep diaries are usually kept for at least 1 to 2 weeks in order to recognize a pattern in the child's sleep habits.

In a clinical setting besides typical sleep duration measurement, sleep diaries can help us understand child sleep problem and also identify areas of inconsistency. Sleep diary, together with sleep questionnaire, is a critical tool in evaluating child's sleep habits.[8] Sleep diaries are frequently used also in treatment outcome research to document intervention effect. They are likewise indispensable in preparation for certain specialized sleep studies, enhancing their validity by showing stable child's sleep patterns in the preparation of the study.

Sleep diaries are frequently used in conjunction with other more objective methods such as actigraphy to control the quality of the actigraphic data and aid in their scoring.[9,10] Pediatric actigraphic studies usually rely on sleep diaries completed by the parents for detecting externally induced motion and motionless wakefulness that actigraphic algorithms cannot discriminate from sleep.[9,10]

Advantages

Sleep diaries are easy to use and cost-effective. They measure sleep prospectively avoiding the limitations of retrospective self- or parent-reported sleep such as recency effects and recall biases.[8,11] Combined with sleep questionnaires they often provide a good insight in child's sleep habits, enabling the diagnosis of behavior or other type of insomnia or certain parasomnias and other sleep disorders without the need for any additional objective measurements. They are usually in good agreement with more objective measures such as actigraphy as well as polysomnography (PSG) for sleep schedule measures, but the agreement rate is relatively low when sleep quality measures are considered.[8] Recently, across development the growing disagreement between actigraphy and parental reports have been found for some aspects of sleep such as infant nocturnal wakefulness.[11]

Limitations

Main limitation of sleep diaries in infants and small children is that they are usually filled-in by their parents. Parental reports are limited to the extent of their awareness of children's sleep behavior. Although their reports on their child's sleep schedule are quite reliable, the validity drops when it comes to sleep quality measures.[12–14] The discrepancy between parental report about nocturnal wake time and actigraphically determined wakefulness seems to be even more pronounced in children with sleep disorders.[15,16]

As already shown in actigraphic studies, parents are often inconsistent; thus filling in the diaries for extended periods could lead to compliance issues that may compromise the validity of the results.[12,14] Numerous types of sleep diaries are used in clinical practice and research, and similarly to sleep questionnaires there is a striking lack of their psychometric evaluation.[17] Currently, there is no "consesus" diary and almost every pediatric sleep centre uses their own version of sleep diary that are in most intances still in paper form.

Sleep Questionnaires

Sleep questionnaires are another important subjective instrument that can be used in conjunction with sleep diary for assessing sleep and sleep problems in children. They can be used to obtain extensive information on sleep patterns, sleep habits, daytime sleepiness, breathing difficulties, parasomnias, or other sleep-related behaviors. They are a useful tool in clinical and research studies focusing on sleep duration and schedule as well as sleep-related behavior and interaction.[9]

Similarly to sleep diaries, sleep questionnaires can be self-reported or parental-reported instruments. Research has shown that self-reported sleep habits are reliable in high school children.[18] There is, however, evidence to suggest that children as young as 8 years can provide reliable, valid, and meaningful reports of their own health when developmentally appropriate assessment methods are applied.[19,20]

Most questionnaires are age specific.[21] Sleep questionnaires for infants and toddlers usually address the issue of bedtime routines and parental-child interactions around bedtime. In prepubertal children the instruments focus more on sleep-wake patterns, sleep hygiene, routines, and the screening for specific sleep disorders. Toward adolescence more questions relating to sleepiness, sleep-wake rhythm, and emotional well-being are included.

These instruments are vastly a screening tool for healthy population and are less diagnostic tools for specific clinical populations. Their main goal is gathering unbiased information about child's sleep. They are, however, not meant to replace clinical assessment by a sleep specialist. Thus, the best outcome in child' sleep evaluation can be achieved from questionnaires in conjunction with a detailed history and clinical examination.[21]

Advantages

Sleep questionnaires are readily available instruments that do not require special technical equipment. Besides information about sleep duration and sleep schedule they offer a very efficient and cost-effective way for subjective experience of sleep quality and sleep hygiene.

Most of the questionnaires reflect an appraisal of the frequency of sleep complaints. They are usually restricted to a specified time frame that is longer than merely an overnight study. These methods also save time and empower the parents to verbalize their children's sleep problems. Although being subjective, they can provide data about bedtime behaviors that cannot be acquired by more objective methods such as actigraphy (ie, parental soothing behaviors).[9]

Limitations

Many studies have developed tailored questionnaires and Spruyt and Gozal in their thorough review[17] collected an extensive list of published and unpublished pediatric sleep questionnaires and assessed them basing on the fundamental operational principles of instrument development. These instruments generally combined sleep-wake patterns and sleep problems assessment, and several distinct scales were created for sleepiness, circadian preference, sleep-disordered breathing, insomnia, and dreams recollection.[17] As the investigators emphasized, most of the pediatric sleep questionnaires were not validated and standardized using appropriate psychometric criteria, which represent the most serious limitation for their use. Almost 10 years later there are only few standardized pediatric sleep questionnaires, and most tools for specific disease populations are still needed.[22] It is encouraging, however, that there are more published normative values and more studies with at least some psychometric validation.[22] There is also increasing recognition for disease-specific instruments or instruments for specific populations.[22]

The retrospective nature of the questionnaires that are usually restricted to a specific time frame renders them to be biased due to recall issues. Thus, they are less accurate for the assessment of some sleep parameters than sleep diaries.[9] Most questionnaires are generic in content and are parental reports. It has been, however, suggested that self-reported questionnaires, especially in school-aged children, might provide complementary information that would not be covered if only relying on parental reports.[23] As children get older, parents may not be aware of their later bedtimes, difficulties falling asleep, night wakings and poor sleep quality, or other certain aspects of children' s sleep hygiene. Thus, the description of child's sleep by the parents seems appropriate as far as symptoms are concerned, but they are less correct in estimating sleep onset or sleep duration.[24]

Additional limitation of the pediatric sleep questionnaires is also that they mostly focus on night sleep and only a few of them incorporate also napping behavior.[17]

OBJECTIVE METHODS
Behavioral Observation and Videosomnography

Assessing sleep in infants and young children is a challenging task. Objective methods of sleep measurement often require sophisticated devices with multiple sensors that can be very obtrusive for a small child. Therefore, it is not surprising that technique of direct behavioral observation has mostly been used to assess sleep in young infants.

Anders and colleagues developed scales for staging sleep in infants based solely on behavioral observations.[25] They argued that particular combinations of behaviors more reliably identified sleep and wake states and even their developmental trajectory than measurement of brain activity via electroencephalogram (EEG). The method of behavioral observation has good interrater reliability for sleep-state scoring in infants and young children and can provide rich information on sleep and wakefulness states and related behaviors.[9] The main advantage is that it can be performed at infant's home. It is, however, very labor intensive and rarely performed overnight. It requires trained observer who complete real-time scoring of sleep and wakefulness states usually in a limited period during daytime.

Anders and Sostek[26] therefore developed videosomnography based on video recordings of sleeping children that can be done in the natural sleep environment and provide whole-night recordings of sleep patterns. It can additionally document parental intervention and the child's behavior during night wakings. Home videos can be used also to document different episodes, reported by parents at clinical evaluation for parasomnias or other nocturnal events. It has been reported that videosomnography can even screen apneas.[27] The limitations include the need for home installation of the recording equipment and for some parents even the feeling of compromised privacy.[9]

Actigraphy

Actigraphy is an objective method for estimation of habitual sleep-wake patterns from activity levels. It consists of continuous monitoring of activity with a watch-shaped movement sensor, attached to different parts of the body. The recommended placement of the actigraph is on the nondominant wrist for older children and adolescents and on the ankle or calf for infants and toddlers.[28]

Because of its nonobtrusiveness actigraphy is frequently used in pediatric clinical and research setting where it can be used for activity measurement over prolonged periods.[28–30] American Academy of Sleep Medicine (AASM) in its updated standards and practice parameters recommend the use of actigraphy in the assessment of pediatric patients with insomnia or circadian rhythm disorders and to monitor total sleep time before testing with the multiple sleep latency test in pediatric patients with suspected central disorders of hypersomnolence.[31] Actigraphy can be highly valuable stand-alone or complementary assessment tool for the evaluation in clinical complaints of excessive daytime sleepiness, prolonged sleep onset latency, multiple and/or prolonged night wakings, and restless sleep.[32] It may provide

additional information above and beyond subjective history, especially when the results of PSG are abnormal or inconclusive. Differential diagnoses that may be seen with actigraphy thus include poor sleep hygiene, irregular sleep patterns, insufficient sleep, and poor sleep quality or low sleep efficiency. It can be used also for documenting treatment response in children with sleep disorders.[32]

Studies in children and adolescents have shown a loss of up to 30% of weekly actigraphic recordings due to illness, technical problems, and/or participant noncompliance.[6] Thus, studies aiming to collect 5 nights of actigraphic data should likely record the activity for at least a week. Individual differences in sleep period and sleep duration likely require more than 7 nights of recording. Thus, from a practical point, especially in the evaluation of circadian sleep-wake rhythm disorders, actigraphic data should be collected for 2 or 3 weeks.

Actigraphy is also a very valuable tool in infant sleep research,[33] although there are no standards in actigraphy sleep scoring rules (for review see Meltzer and colleagues[30]). Actigraphy can be used to distinguish between sleep-disturbed and control infants and also to assess the efficacy of behavioral sleep interventions.[12,34] During the first year of life even active and quiet sleep can be identified with reasonable validity.[35]

There are numerous types of actigraphic devices that are usually small and lightweight but differ in technical specifications and modes of operation and data collection, therefore rendering their comparison difficult. Because of lack of standard scoring rules and variable definitions, Meltzer and colleagues[30] suggested rules for reporting of actigraphy in pediatric sleep research. The latter can be useful also for clinical practice. The same group recently also provided comprehensive reference values for pediatric actigraphy, based on a very large sample of healthy school-aged children and adolescents.[36] Similar reference values for infants and toddlers are still missing. Therefore, it is important to interpret the results in the proper context, by comparison with other studies that used similar devices and technical specifications.

Advantages

Actigraphy offers relatively inexpensive way to collect naturalistic sleep data of a child in his home environment over multiple consecutive days up to several weeks. Therefore, it is particularly suitable for the assessment of sleep in longitudinal studies along multiple assessment points. There it provides more objective measure than parental reports, which can limit the range and accuracy of information about the child's sleep.[15,16]

Limitations

The assessment of sleep and wakefulness from activity levels offers only estimation of the true sleep-wake patterns and does not discriminate between the different sleep stages. Ever since Sadeh developed first algorithm for validly identifying sleep and wake in healthy infants,[37] multiple algorithms have been developed for different types of devices and research groups.[30] However, many actigraphic algorithms have not been validated for specific ages and/or disease populations in children.[38,39]

The notable finding in the review by Meltzer and colleagues[30] is the consistent report of poor specificity in pediatric actigraphic studies across all age groups and devices, thus revealing limited ability of actigraphy to accurately detect wake after sleep onset among pediatric populations. Actigraphy is therefore not a suitable method for the diagnosis of disorders in which sleep is fragmented.[40]

Actigraphy is also prone to artifacts from externally induced motion and motionless wakefulness that actigraphic algorithms cannot discriminate from sleep.[9] Therefore, one of the main challenges is the need of parental adherence to complete 24-hour sleep-wake diaries over several consecutive days.[41]

Polysomnography

In-laboratory attended PSG is the gold standard or so-called type 1 (level 1) sleep study for diagnosing sleep disorders and can be performed in children of all ages. Its unattended variant, which includes 7 or more channels and can be recorder in outpatient setting in more naturalistic home environment, is classified as type 2 study (for recent review see Arnardottir and colleagues[2]).

In an ideal setting pediatric in-laboratory full-night PSG should consist up to 12 hours of sleep in a quiet, darkened room with an ambient temperature of around 22°C, in the company of one of the parents.[42] Six to eight channels of EEG with bilateral electrooculogram and chin electromyogram (EMG) consist essential features for sleep stage scoring. Multiple additional parameters need to be measured according to the patient's suspected disorder.[43] Standard respiratory parameters include measurement of respiratory flow, respiratory effort, and arterial oxygen saturation. Airflow can be assessed via an oronasal thermistor and/or nasal cannula. It is highly recommended to use multiple measurements of airflow due to the frequent loss of the signal caused by secretions, suckling artifact, or displacement of the sensor.

In pediatric PSG it is crucial to include a sensor for oral breathing because many children with sleep-disordered breathing have an enlarged adenoid and breath through their mouth.[42] Therefore after the neonatal period thermistors with joint nasal and oral probes are used for that purpose. The preferred method for the evaluation of respiratory effort is chest and abdominal respiratory inductance plethysmography that is typically used in the uncalibrated mode to avoid repetition of calibration procedure after body movements.[42] Other possible sensors for respiratory effort assessment include piezoelectric belts, intercostal EMG, and esophageal pressure monitoring. Arterial oxygen saturation (SpO2) is commonly performed by pulse oximetry. Monitoring of the pulse waveform in addition to saturation value might be helpful in distinguishing true desaturations from motion artifacts that are frequent in child's sleep.[42] Respiratory flow can be measured also using a sidestream end-tidal capnography. Carbon dioxide (CO_2) measurements are recommended as an important parameter in pediatric sleep studies for quantitative measurement of hypoventilation. Children with obstructive sleep apnea have frequently partial airway obstructions, and oxygen desaturations are less common than in adults.[44] It is therefore important that PSG evaluation of children with possible sleep breathing disorders includes end-tidal or transcutaneous CO_2 measurement to evaluate nocturnal hypoventilation.[44] Leg movements for diagnosing periodic limb movement disorder or supporting the diagnosis of restless legs syndrome are assessed by bilateral anterior tibial EMG. They can be seen also via digital time-synchronized video recording that can be extremely helpful in the assessment of parasomnias, seizures, and unusual respiratory events.[42] Body position can be assessed also through an analog output from body position sensor. Recording in laboratory includes also audio recording that can detect snoring. The latter is usually assessed via tracheal sound monitored with a microphone sensor or indirectly assessed from airflow sensor. PSG recordings also include an electrocardiogram (ECG).

In-laboratory PSG is currently accepted as gold standard for diagnosing sleep-disordered breathing in children.[45,46] According to AASM practice parameters PSG is also a standard method for diagnosing periodic limb movement disorder and evaluation for suspected narcolepsy.[47] It has to be performed before multiple sleep latency test (MSLT) in the evaluation of excessive somnolence and to quantify sleepiness. Nonrespiratory indications for PSG in children include also children with frequent or an atypical or potentially injurious parasomnia, epilepsy, or other spells to be differentiated from parasomnia or nocturnal enuresis, who should be clinically screened for comorbid sleep-disordered breathing or periodic limb movement disorder.[47]

Advantages

PSG recordings provide reliable, unbiased, and objective information about a variety of sleep-related events, such as disturbance in respiratory parameters and sleep architecture. The overall approach to sleep scoring is similar to that in adults; however, pediatric-specific scoring rules include sleep staging for infants and scoring rules for apneas and hypopneas.[48] In children aged 5 years and older, besides PSG, MSLT is also technically feasible that has been recognized as a valid tool for objective evaluation of daytime sleepiness.[47,49] However, there are currently no widely acceptable MSLT norms for children, especially in preschool children who nap regularly.[50]

Limitations

Despite PSG being the gold standard for diagnosing sleep disorders, it can be quite challenging in pediatrics because of children's limited ability for cooperation in the setup and troubles with sleeping in the laboratory environment; this is especially true in younger children and children with different neurodevelopmental problems. In-laboratory recording is also very expensive and time- and labor-consuming. It requires appropriate technical equipment and skilled professional staff to ensure the quality of the study and in many places it is therefore not readily available. Thus, most clinical and research sleep studies are typically only applied for a single night. This represents a major limitation of PSG, because night-to-night variability in different sleep parameters and the potential first night effect of sleeping with a device are not measured. Unfamiliar environment, discomfort, and limitation of the movement due to the attached electrodes can reduce sleep quality in the laboratory setting, which is known as the so called first night effect.[51] It has been shown that infants do not display a first night effect.[52] However, older children have more pronounced first night effect mainly for parameters related to rapid eye movement (REM) sleep such as prolongation of the REM sleep and REM sleep latency on the second night of the recording.[53,54] There is, however, less agreement for other parameters such as sleep onset latency and sleep efficiency.[55]

Home Sleep Apnea Testing

Because of known limitations of PSG, in recent years, there has been increased interest in less obtrusive methods that would allow objective sleep assessment in children in more naturalistic home environment. Home sleep apnea testing (HSAT) is of considerable interest, as it has the potential to measure a more typical night's sleep in a child, could be substantially less expensive, and therefore potentially accessible to more children.

HSATs are type 2 and 3 studies that can be performed in ambulatory setting and typically use fewer sensors than PSG. Type 3 sleep study is also called polygraphy (PG), portable monitroring, or cardiorespiratory study.[48]

Unattended PSG is a type 2 study that has the advantage of a home-based complete sleep study allowing the diagnosis of sleep-disordered breathing and also numerous nonrespiratory sleep disorders. However, in children there are no randomized controlled trials, and the information on pediatric unattended home PSG is limited.[42,56] In healthy school-aged children it has been demonstrated that it is feasible to obtain high-quality PSG at child's home but clearly more research especially in younger children and children with more restless sleep is needed.[57–59]

Direct comparison of in-laboratory and home PSG has shown that children sleep longer in the home environment with a trend to more consolidated sleep.[58] However, the hook-up process must be performed by a trained sleep technician. Unattended PSG is therefore still labor and time intensive and also relatively expensive. No portable PSG includes any video recording that often might provide useful information, especially in evaluating parasomnias, nocturnal epilepsy, or other complex nocturnal behaviors. Home CO_2 monitoring is also less commonly available in ambulatory PSG, thus not allowing detection of obstructive alveolar hypoventilation.

Most of the HSAT studies in children have used type 3 multichannel polygraphic devices that usually measure multiple respiratory parameters such as airflow, respiratory effort, and arterial oxygen saturation. In addition, some include also ECG, pulse wave, and body position assessment. Type 3 devices with limited channels, however, lack measurement of actual sleep and therefore do not provide data regarding total sleep time. Because these devices measure fewer physiologic variables than PSG, they may lead to underestimation of the presence or severity of disease.[60] In pediatric obstructive sleep apnea (OSA) partial airway obstruction is more common and oxygen desaturation less common in comparison to adults.[44] Therefore, HSATs without EEG recording and absence of CO_2 measurement would miss hypopnea causing arousals and/or obstructive hypoventilation. Severity of OSA may be underestimated also in a poor night's sleep recording with reduced REM sleep, because obstructive upper airway events in children tend to cluster during REM sleep.[61] One of the disadvantages of home studies is also the risk of failed study due to movement of the sensors or signal loss. The signal most at risk for disruption is the nasal flow signal.[61] Under carefully controlled conditions with electrode placement by trained staff, however, HSAT may be technically feasible even in young preschool children.[60] There are limited published validation data comparing HSAT with the gold standard of PSG in children. Despite discordant results, sensitivity and specificity of home PSG seem to be reasonably good for the diagnosis of moderate and severe OSA in children who have a high pretest probability of having the condition.[61] There are, however, no validation studies for the use of HSAT in infants and toddlers or children with comorbid medical condition in whom misdiagnosing or underdiagnosing is potentially more severe. Therefore, the AASM task force on HSATs for the diagnosis of OSA in children noted that there were insufficient data to support using HSATs for the diagnosis of OSA in children.[60] But nevertheless they recommend continuing development and validation of HSAT devices for this population.

Oximetry

The least extensive sleep studies are type 4 studies, which include only 1 or 2 channels, with oximetry usually being used as one of the measurements. Oximetry commonly measures oxygen saturation in the blood via pulse oximetry. Nocturnal oximetry has long been proposed as a screening tool for pediatric OSA due to its reliability, simplicity, and suitability for children.[62,63] A positive oximetry result indicates moderate-to-severe OSA, and in this case PSG does not seem to be required for adenotonsillectomy referral.[64] Its sensitivity is, however, low and if oximetry recording is abnormal or inconclusive, the clinical suspicion of OSA should be assessed by nocturnal PSG.[65] Oximetry can namely miss some obstructive breathing without desaturation.[65]

Overnight oximetry is thus a valuable, low-cost, and easy tool to identify severe OSA. It can be performed in home environment and allows for multiple night recording. Pulse oximetry can be interfaced with a smartphone, increasing the portability of the device.[65,66] However, only a few studies have critically examined the distribution of nocturnal oximetry values in healthy children for subsequently defining criteria for pathologic

values and severity range.[67] Therefore, oximetry alone is certainly not adequate for the universal diagnosis of OSA in children.[60,61]

FUTURE POTENTIALS

Although in-laboratory PSG stays the gold standard for the evaluation of sleep and sleep disorders in children due to its complexity, it might not be readily available for all children with expanding frequency of sleep disorders. In pediatric OSA it has been shown that PSG criteria alone or in combination with the patient history and physical examination often do not suffice for accurate diagnosis and particularly its severity.[68] PSG is also poorly predictive of OSA-associated morbidities.[68] On the other hand, not every snoring child with large tonsils needs to be referred for a tertiary level sleep consultation. The rationale in sleep assessment should therefore be a combination of several criteria, from the presence of specific symptoms and/or biomarkers related to OSA, to the use of PSG measures with consensus-derived cut-off values and additional incorporation of measurable outcomes. So designed algorithms could improve the recognition of those clinically referred children who would most likely benefit from treatment.[69] Alternatively, novel unbiased diagnostic approaches that are both sensitive and specific, require less effort, and are more affordable need to be identified to permit prospective screening of the large number of habitually snoring children.

One of such approaches could be noninvasive assessment of changes in autonomic nervous system tone with addition of other relatively nonobtrusive sensor technologies that record oxygen saturation, snoring, body position, airflow, and actigraphy.[69] Although measurements of central nervous system signals is considered superior and is most common for sleep analyses in general, both sleep and sleep-disordered breathing could be accurately and reliably assessed based on changes in autonomic signals.[56]

Autonomic Signal Assessment

One of such signals is *heart rate variability (HRV)*, a well-established technique for studying the modulatory effects of neural mechanisms on the sinus node with 2 major components, high and low frequency, that change with age and sleep stage.[70] Assessing HRV may provide some indications regarding the general quantity and quality of sleep,[56,71] and it has been shown that moderate to severe childhood OSA is associated with HRV changes.[72,73] Some researchers found that measuring pulse rate variability by pulse plethysmography is even more accurate than HRV for the detection of sleep apnea,[74] suggesting that peripheral pulse measurement is preferred over ECG measurements. However, more research is needed before these methods could be validated for clinical use in children with sleep disorders.

Measurement of the peripheral blood flow is the basis of the novel technique based on autonomic signals, the *peripheral arterial tonometry (PAT)*. The PAT signal measures the finger's arterial pulsatile volume changes by a unique plethysmography that reflect sympathetic nervous system activities.[75] The PAT device, which is usually combined with pulse rate, oxygen saturation, and actigraphy measurements, indirectly detects apnea and hypopnea events by identifying surges of sympathetic activation associated with the termination of respiratory events. There are some published studies using this system in children that showed that PAT device can detect autonomic arousals,[76] being superior to oximetry in detecting children with sleep-disordered breathing.[77] Direct comparison of PAT device with PSG in laboratory recording recently showed excellent agreement between the 2 methods in apnea-hypopnea index measurement,[78,79] suggesting PAT can be a reasonably suitable method to detect sleep stages and OSA at least in adolescents. In children, however, clearly more data are needed.

Another useful methodology assessing autonomic function is the *pulse transit time (PTT)*. PTT refers to the time a pulse wave takes to travel between the heart and the periphery and therefore requires the measurement of ECG and pulse. The speed at which this arterial pressure wave travels is directly proportional to blood pressure. Although mainly used in research setting, the PTT can, similarly to PAT, serve as a noninvasive marker for autonomic arousals. Their measurements may be specifically valuable in children because upper airway obstructive events in children frequently terminate without visible cortical arousals.[80] Several studies have shown that PTT in children is a valuable method for detecting microarousals and respiratory-related autonomic arousals.[81,82] Recent meta-analysis of 21 pediatric PTT studies, besides its usefulness in detecting obstructive events, revealed also a potential of PTT to detect central apneic events in infants and children.[83] Thus, in the future the method could be used also for clinical purposes. However, its main limitation is the high percentage of the artifacts.[84]

Electroencephalogram Analysis

Conventional methods for assessing the disruption of sleep quality involve visual scoring of the EEG and an assessment of sleep architecture.

New technologies and computers have revolutionized our views of how to monitor and how to interpret the monitoring of physiologic functions during sleep. The analytical window in any automated sleep system is much shorter than basing of a visual scoring. However, clinical visual scoring can distinguish cortical arousals from subcortical activations,[85] although there is not enough evidence regarding clinical significance of the latter.[86] Unlike in adults, sleep architecture in children with sleep-disordered breathing is often relatively preserved with only about half of apneic events terminating with cortical arousal as defined by adult criteria.[86] Spectral analysis of EEG may therefore provide a more sensitive measure of sleep disruption at respiratory event termination in children with sleep disordered breathing than conventional sleep architecture or arousal indices.[56] Besides spectral EEG analysis several different sleep EEG measures have been assessed in basic and clinical research in the course of development, with their discrepancies indicating neurodevelopmental disorders.[40] These measures include the percentage of REM and slow wave sleep, the slope of sleep slow waves, sleep spindle characteristics as well as EEG coherence measurements.

Wearables and Smartphone Applications

Technological advancement led to the development of different consumer-wearable devices and smartphone applications that can potentially assess sleep via movement detection and/or diverse biosignals such as pulse or heart rate or oximetry. Although being easy to use and allowing monitoring in home environment, these activity trackers indicated high validity for steps, distance, and energy expenditure measurements but much lower validity for sleep estimation.[87] In children and adolescents these commercially available devices are less explored or validated, not rendering them as appropriate surrogate for validated actigraphs.[39] Likewise, only few studies evaluated smartphone applications in children and usually found no correlation between total sleep time or sleep latency between app and PSG.[88] However, by a specific placement of a smartphone enabling pulse sensing much better correlation of sleep parameters can be achieved.[89] It has been already suggested that pulse oximeter integrated with a smartphone could help in screening children with sleep disordered breathing.[90] Thus, with enabling additional signals sensing, such as snoring sounds and movements, as well as improved algorithms, there might be a future potential for these devices to be a reasonable substitution for sleep and sleep quality measurements in children and adults.[56]

Biomarkers

Novel technologies, such as genomics, proteomics, lipidomics, or metabolomics, allow exploration of unique expression of certain genes or proteins in specific sleep disorders.[91,92] These methods could identify presence or absence of specific biomarkers or a particular cluster of markers closely linked to sleep disorder diagnosis or associated end-organ morbidity. Such biomarkers could help in designing specific algorithms for population screening and potentially enable priority assignment for treatment and outcome monitoring in those children considered at increased risk.[69] In pediatric OSA several biomarkers aimed at the diagnosis or detection of OSA-related morbidities have been explored but are not necessarily implemented by all sleep practitioners.[91,93] However, the usability of other biomarkers in clinical practice is often limited, as no references for normal ranges of metabolites exist.[92]

SUMMARY

Sleep plays a critical role in the development of healthy children. Detecting sleep and sleep disorders and the effectiveness of interventions for improving sleep in children require valid sleep measures. Assessment of sleep in children, in particular infants and young children, can be a quite challenging task. Although in-laboratory full-night PSG remains the gold standard for the evaluation of sleep and sleep disorders in children and adolescents, this complex method is not the right tool for every sleep problem and might not be readily accessible.

Many subjective and objective methods are available to evaluate various aspects of sleep in childhood, each with their strengths and limitations. None can, however, replace the importance of thorough clinical interview with detailed history and clinical examination by a sleep specialist.

Technological advancement enabled development of less complex but still reliable tools for less obtrusive sleep measurements in child's naturalistic home environment. However, given the fact that different assessment methods may yield different results, a combination of different instruments often provides best insight in child's sleep and its disorders. Together with evolving biomarkers, these combinations might help in designing algorithms for better recognition of those clinically referred children who would most likely benefit from treatment.

Novel technologies and the increased awareness of the public on the importance of sleep and sleep disorders led to the development of simple devices that with some future improvements and additional clinical research might hold a potential for surrogate sleep assessment.

CLINICS CARE POINTS

- Sleep diaries or sleep logs are easy to use and cost-effective tool for tracking sleep and documenting sleep problem. Together with sleep questionnaires are, despite being subjective, a critical tool in evaluating child's sleep habits. They represent a good screening tool to be used before the first visit to a sleep specialist.

- Despite numerous different pediatric sleep questionnaires only few have been validated and standardized using appropriate psychometric criteria. Sleep questionnaires are age specific and there is increasing recognition for disease-specific questionnaires or instruments for specific populations.

- Actigraphy provides relatively inexpensive method for more objective estimation of habitual sleep-wake patterns. Due to its non-obtrusiveness it is particularly usefull in pediatric clinical and research setting. It can be used for the evaluation in clinical complaints of excessive daytime sleepiness, insomnia or circadian rhythm disorders.

- In-laboratory attended full-night polysomnography remains the gold standard for diagnosing sleep disorders and can be performed in children of all ages.

- Home sleep apnea testing provides less obtrusive method that can be used to measure a more typical night's sleep in a child in his home environment. It allows detection of sleep disordered breathing and can be used as a screening tool. However, it must be taken into account that it may underestimate the presence or severity of sleep disordered breathing.

- Several biomarkers may be useful when evaluating sleep conditions in children in the clinical practice. However, only a combination of different instruments together with thoroug clinical interview and physical exam provides the best insight in the child's sleep and its disorders.

DISCLOSURE

The author has nothing to disclose.

REFERENCES

1. Jiang F. Sleep and Early Brain Development. Ann Nutr Metab 2019;75(suppl1):44–53.
2. Arnardottir SE, Islind AS, Óskarsdóttir M. The future of sleep measurements: a review and perspctive. Sleep Med Clin 2021;16:447–64.
3. Roffwarg HP, Muzio JN, Dement WC. Ontogenetic development of the human sleep-dream cycle. Science 1966;152:604–19.
4. Buysee DJ, Anconi-Israel S, Edinger JD, et al. Recommendations for standard research assesment of insomnia. Sleep 2006;29:1155–73.
5. Harrison EM, Yablonsky AM, Powell AL, et al. Reported light is the sleep environment: enhancement of the sleep diary. Nat Sci Sleep 2019;11:11–26.
6. Accebo C, Sadeh A, Seifer R, et al. Estimating sleep patterns with activity monitoring in children and adolescents: how many nights are necessary for reliable measures? Sleep 1999;22:95–103.
7. Moore M, Kirchner HL, Drotar D, et al. Correlates of adolescent sleep time and variability in sleep time: the role of individual and health related characteristics. Sleep Med 2011;12:239–45.
8. Short MA, Arora T, Gradisar M, et al. How many sleep diary entries are needed to reliable estimate adolescent sleep? Sleep 2017;40:zsx006.
9. Sadeh A. Sleep assesment methods. Monogr Soc Res Child Dev 2015;80:33–84.
10. Tétreault E, Bélanger ME, Bernier A, et al. Actigraphy data in pediatric research: the role of sleep diaries. Sleep Med 2018;47:86–92.
11. Tikotzky L, Volkovich E. Infant nocturnal wakefulness: a longitudinal study comparing three sleep assessment methods. Sleep 2019;42:1–12.
12. Sadeh A. Assessment of intervention for infant night waking: parental reports and activity-based home monitroing. J Consult Clin Psychol 1994;62:63–8.
13. Tikotzky L, Sadeh A. Maternal sleep-related cognition and infant sleep: a longitudinal study from pregnancy through the first year. Child Dev 2009;80:860–74.
14. Werner H, Molinari L, Guyer C, et al. Agreement rates between actigraphy, diary, and questionnaire for children's sleep patterns. Arch Pediatr Adolesc Med 2008;162:350–8.
15. Kushnir J, Sadeh A. Correspondence between reported and actigraphic sleep measures in preschool children: the role of a clinical context. J Clin Sleep Med 2013;9:1147–51.
16. Werner H, Hunkeler P, Benz C, et al. Valid methods for estimating children's sleep problems in clinical practice. Acta Pediatr 2014;103:e555–7.
17. Spruyt K, Gozal D. Pediatric sleep questionnaires as diagnostic or epidemiological tools: a review of currently available instruments. Sleep Med Rev 2011;15:19–32.
18. Gaina A, Sekine M, Chen XL, et al. Validity of child sleep diary questionnaire among junior high school children. J Epidemiol 2004;14:1–4.
19. Eaden J, Mayberry JF. Questionnaires: the use and abuse of social survey methods in medical research. Postgrad Med J 1999;75:397–400.
20. Riley AW. Evidence that school-age children can self report on their health. Ambul Pediatr 2004;4:371–6.
21. AlNabhani A, Shapiro CM. Survey tools and screening questionnaires in pediatric sleep medicine. In: Gozal D, Kheirandish-Gozal L, editors. Pediatric sleep medicine. Mechanisms and comprehensive guide to clinical evaluation and management. Cham (Switzerland): Springer; 2021. p. 135–58.
22. Sen T, Spruyt K. Pediatric sleep tools: an updated literature review. Front Psychiatry 2020;11:317.
23. Meltzer LJ, Avis KT, Biggs S, et al. The Children's Report of Sleep Patterns (CRSP): a self-report measure of sleep for school-age children. J Clin Sleep Med 2013;9:235–45.
24. Dayyat EA, Spruyt K, Molfese DL, et al. Sleep estimates in children: parental versus actigraphic assessment. Nat Sci Sleep 2011;3:115–23.
25. Anders TF, Keener M. Developmental course of nighttime sleep-wake patterns in full-term and premature infants during the first year of life. I. Sleep 1985;8:173–92.
26. Anders TF, Sostek AM. The use of time lapsed video recording of sleep-wake behavior in human infants. Psychophysiology 1976;13:155–8.
27. Sivan Y, Kornecki A, Schonfeld T. Screening obstructive apnea syndrome by home videotape recording in children. Eur Respir J 1996;9:2127–31.
28. Sadeh A, Acebo C. The role and validity of actigraphy in sleep medicine. Sleep Med Rev 2002;6:113–24.
29. Sadeh A. The role and validity of actigraphy in sleep medicine: an update. Sleep Med Rev 2011;15:259–67.
30. Meltzer LJ, Montgomery-Downs HE, Insana SP, et al. Use of actigraphy for asessment in pediatric sleep research. Sleep Med Rev 2012;16:463–75.
31. Smith MT, McCrae CS, Cheung J, et al. Use of actigraphy for the eveluation of sleep disorders and circadian rhythm sleep-wake disorders: an American Academy of Sleep Medicine clinical practice guideline. J Clin Sleep Med 2018;14:1231–7.
32. Montgomery-Downs HE, Tikotzky L. Actigraphy. In: Gozal D, Kheirandish-Gozal L, editors. Pediatric sleep medicine. Mechanisms and comprehensive guide to clinical evaluation and management. Cham (Switzerland): Springer; 2021. p. 271–82.

33. Gnidovec B, Naubauer D, Zidar J. Actigraphic assessment of sleep-wake rhythm during the first 6 months of life. Clin Neurophysiol 2002;113:1815–21.

34. Sadeh A. Evaluating night wakings in sleep-disturbed infants: a methodological study of parental reports and actigraphy. Sleep 1996;19:757–62.

35. Sadeh A, Acebo C, Seifer R, et al. Activity-based assessment of sleep-wake patterns during the 1st year of life. Infant Behav Dev 1995;18:329–37.

36. Meltzer LJ, Short M, Booster GD, et al. Pediatric motor activity during sleep as measured by actigraphy. Sleep 2019;42:zsy196.

37. Sadeh A, Lavie P, Scher A, et al. Actigraphic home-monitoring sleep-disturbed and control infants and young children: a new method for pediatric assesment of sleep-wake patterns. Pediatrics 1991;78:494–9.

38. Cole RJ, Kripke DF, Gruen W, et al. Automatic sleep wake identification from wrist activity. Sleep 1992;15:461–9.

39. Meltzer LJ, Walsh CM, Traylor J, et al. Direct comparison of two new actigraphs and polysomnography in children and adolescents. Sleep 2012;35:159–66.

40. Mouthon AL, Huber R. Methods in pediatric sleep research and sleep medicine. Neuropediatrics 2015;46:159–70.

41. Galland B, Meredith-Jones K, Terrill P, et al. Challenges and emerging technology within the field of pediatric actigraphy. Front Psychiatry 2014;5:99.

42. Beck SE, Marcus CL. Pediatric polysomnography. Sleep Med Clin 2009;4:393–406.

43. Iber C, Ancoli-Israel S, Chesson A, et al, editors. The AASM manual of the scoring of sleep and associated events: rules, terminology and technical specifications. 1st edition. Westcheser (NY): American Academy of Sleep Medicine; 2007. p. 1–59.

44. Gozal D, Capdevila OS, Kheirandish-Gozal L. Metabolic alterations and systemic inflammation in obstuctive sleep apnea among nonobese and obese prepubertal children. Am J Respir Crit Care Med 2008;177:369–75.

45. Marcus CL, Brooks LJ, Draper KA, et al. American Academy of Pedaitrics. Diagnosing and management of childhood obstructive sleep apnea syndrome. Pedaitrics 2012;130:576–84.

46. Aurora NR, Zak RS, Karippot A, et al. Practice parameters for respiratory indications for polysomnography in children. Sleep 2011;34:379–88.

47. Aurora NR, Lamm CI, Zak RS, et al. Practice parameters for non-respiratory indications for polysomnography and multiple sleep latency testing for children. Sleep 2012;35:1467–73.

48. Berry RB, Brooks R, Gamaldo CE, et al. The AASM manual for the scoring of sleep and associated events: rules, terminology and technical specifications, Version 2.6. Darien (IL): American Academy of Sleep Medicine.; 2020.

49. Kotagal S, Nichols CD, Grigg-Damberger MM, et al. Non-respiratory indications for polysomnography and selected procedures in children: an evidence based review. Sleep 2012;35:1451–66.

50. Zhang M, Thieux M, Vieux N, et al. Multiple sleep latency test. In: Gozal D, Kheirandish-Gozal L, editors. Pediatric sleep medicine. Mechanisms and comprehensive guide to clinical evaluation and management. Cham (Switzerland): Springer; 2021. p. 259–70.

51. Agnew HW, Webb WB, Williams RL. The first night effect: an EEG study of sleep. Psychophysiology 1966;2:263–6.

52. Rebuffat E, Groswasser J, Kelmanson I, et al. Polygraphic evaluation of night-to-night variability in sleep characteristic and apneas in infants. Sleep 1994;17:329–32.

53. Scholle S, Scholle HF, Kemper A, et al. First night effect in children and adolescents undergoing polysomnography for sleep-disordered breathing. Clin Neurophysiol 2003;114:2138–45.

54. Li AM, Wing YK, Cheung A, et al. Is a 2-night polysomnographic study necessary in childhood sleep-related disordered breathing? Chest 2004;126:1467–72.

55. Verhulst SL, Schrauwen N, De Backer WA, et al. First night effect for polysomnographic data in children and adolescents with suspected sleep disordered breathing. Arch Dis Child 2006;91:233–7.

56. Etzioni-Friedman T, Pillar GL. Technologies in the pediatric sleep lab: present and future. In: Gozal D, Kheirandish-Gozal L, editors. Pediatric sleep medicine. Mechanisms and comprehensive guide to clinical evaluation and management. Cham (Switzerland): Springer; 2021. p. 179–91.

57. Goodwin JL, Enright PL, Kaemingh KL, et al. Feasibility of using unattended ambulatory polysomnography in children for reserach – report of the Tucson Children's Assessment of Sleep Apnea study (TuCASA). Sleep 2001;24:937–44.

58. Marcus CL, Traylor J, Bradford R, et al. Feasibility of comprehensive unattended home polysomnography in school-aged children. J Clin Sleep Med 2014;10:913–8.

59. Brockmann PE, Perez JL, Moya A. Feasibility of unattended home polysomnography in children with sleep disordered breathing. Int J Pediatr Otorhinolaryngol 2013;77:1960–4.

60. Kirk V, Baughn J, D'Andrea L, et al. American Academy of Sleep Medicine position paper for the use of a home sleep apnea test for the diagnosis of OSA in children. J Clin Sleep Med 2017;13:1199–203.

61. Tan HL, Kheirandish-Gozal L, Gozal D. Pediatric home sleep apnea testing: slowly getting there! Chest 2015;148:1382–95.

62. Brouillette RT, Morielli A, Leimanis A, et al. Nocturnal pulse oximetry as an abbreviated testing modality for pediatric obstructive sleep apnea. Pedaitric 2000;105:405–12.

63. Kaditis A, Kheirandish-Gozal L, Gozal D. Pediatric OSAS: oximetry can provide answers when polysomnography is not available. Sleep Med Rev 2016;27:96–105.

64. Nixon GM, Kermack AS, Davis CM, et al. Planning adenotonsillectomy in children with obstructive sleep apnea: the role of overnight oximetry. Pediatrics 2004;113:19–25.

65. Garde A, Hoppenbrouwer X, Dehkordi P, et al. Pediatric pulse oximetry-based OSA screening at different thresholds of the apnea-hypopnea index with an expression of uncertainity for inconclusive classifications. Sleep Med 2019;60:45–52.

66. Petersen CL, Chen TP, Ansermino JM, et al. Desing and eveluation of a low-cost smartphone pulse oximeter. Sensors (Basel) 2013;13:16882–93.

67. Urschitz MS, Wolff J, Von Einem V, et al. Reference values for nocturnal home oximetry during sleep in primary school children. Chest 2003;123:96–101.

68. Tan HL, Kheirandish-Gozal L, Gozal D. The promise of translational and personalised approaches for paediatric obstructive sleep apnoea: an 'Omics' perspective. Thorax 2014;69:450–6.

69. Kheirandish-Gozal L. What is »abnormal« in pediatric sleep? Respir Care 2010;55:1366–73.

70. Villa MP, Calcagnini G, Pagani J, et al. Effects of sleep stage and age on short-term heart rate variability. Chest 2000;117:460–6.

71. Rodrigez-Colon SM, He F, Bixler EO, et al. Sleep variablity and cardiac autonomic modulation in adolescents – Penn State Child Cohort (PSCC) study. Sleep Med 2015;16:67–72.

72. Walter LM, Nixon GM, Davey MJ, et al. Autonomic dysfunction in children with sleep disordered breathing. Sleep Breath 2013;17:605–12.

73. Nisbet LC, Yiallourou SR, Nixon GM, et al. Nocturnal autonomic function in preschool children with sleep-disordered breathing. Sleep Med 2013;14:1310–6.

74. Lazaro J, Gil E, Vergara JM, et al. Pulse rate variability analysis for discrimination of sleep-apnea-related decreases in the amplitude fluctuations of pulse photoplethysmographic signal in children. IEEE J Biomed Health Inform 2014;18:240–6.

75. Bar A, Pillar G, Dvir I, et al. Evaluation of a portable device based on peripheral atrerial tone for unattended home sleep studies. Chest 2003;123:695–703.

76. Tauman R, O'Brien LM, Mast BT, et al. Peripheral arterial tonometry events and electroencephalographic arousals in children. Sleep 2004;27:502–6.

77. Serra A, Cocuzza S, Maiolino L, et al. The watch-pat in pediatric sleep disordered breathing: pilot study on children with negative nocturnal pulse oximetry. Int J Pediatr Otorhynolaryngol 2017;97:245–50.

78. Tanphaichitr A, Thianboonsong A, Banhiran W, et al. Watch peripheral arterial tonometry in the diagnosis of pediatric obstructive sleep apnea. Otolaryngol Head Neck Surg 2018;159:166–72.

79. Choi JH, Lee B, Lee JY, et al. Validating the watch-PAT for diagnosing obstructive sleep apnea in adolescents. J Clin Sleep Med 2018;14:1741–7.

80. Katz ES, Lutz J, Black C, et al. Pulse transit time as a measure of arousal and respiratory effort in children with sleep disordered breathing. Pediatr Res 2003;53:580–8.

81. Pepin JL, Delavie N, Pin I, et al. Pulse transit time improves detection of sleep respiratory events and microarousals in children. Chest 2005;127:722–30.

82. Brietzke SE, Katz ES, Roberson DW. Pulse transit time as a screening tool for pediatric sleep-related breathing disorders. Arch Otolaryngol Head Neck Surg 2007;133:980–4.

83. Smith LA, Dawes PJ, Galland BC. The use of pulse transit time in pediatric sleep studies: a systematic review. Sleep Med Rev 2018;37:4–13.

84. Griffon L, Amaddeo A, Olmo Arroyo J, et al. Pulse transit time as a tool to characterize obstructive and central apneas in children. Sleep Breath 2018;22:311–6.

85. Grigg-Damberger M, Gozal D, Marcus CL et al. The visual scoring of sleep and arousals in infants and children. J Clin Sleep Med 3:201-40.

86. Yang JSC, Nicholas CL, Nixon GM, et al. EEG spectral analysis of apnoeic events confirming visual scoring in childhood sleep disordered breathing. Sleep Breath 2012;16:491–7.

87. Everson KR, Goto MM, Furberg RD. Systematic review of the validity and realiability of consumer-wearable activity trackers. Int J Behav Nutr Phys Act 2015;12:159.

88. Patel P, Kim JY, Brooks LJ. Accuracy of a smartphone application in estimating sleep in children. Sleep Breath 2017;21:505–11.

89. Toon E, Davey MJ, Hollins SL, et al. Comparison of commercial wrist-based and smartphone accelerometers, actigraphy, and PSG in a clinical cohort of children and adolescents. J Clin Sleep Med 2016;12:343–50.

90. Garde A, Dehkordi P, Karlen W, et al. Development of a screening tool for sleep disordered breathing in children using the phone Oximeter. PLoS One 2014;9:e112959.

91. Kheirandish-Gozal L, Gozal D. Laboratory tests in pediatric sleep medicine. In: Gozal D, Kheirandish-Gozal L, editors. Pediatric sleep medicine. Mechanisms and comprehensive guide to clinical evaluation and management. Cham (Switzerland): Springer; 2021. p. 209–14.

92. Humer E, Pieh C, Brandmayr G. Metabolomics in sleep, indomnia and sleep apnea. Int J Mol Sci 2020;21:7244.

93. Kheirandish-Gozal L, Gozal D. Pediatric OSA syndrome morbidity biomarkers: the hunt is finally on! Chest 2017;151:500–6.

Measuring Sleep, Wakefulness, and Circadian Functions in Neurologic Disorders

Markus H. Schmidt, MD, PhD[a,b,*,1], Martijn P.J. Dekkers, MD, PhD[a,1],
Sébastien Baillieul, MD, PhD[a,c,1], Jasmine Jendoubi, MSc[a,1],
Marie-Angela Wulf, MD, PhD[a,1], Elena Wenz, MD[a,1], Livia Fregolente, MD[a,1],
Albrecht Vorster, PhD[a,1], Oriella Gnarra, MSc[a,d,1],
Claudio L.A. Bassetti, MD[a,e,1]

KEYWORDS

- Sleep • Wakefulness • Circadian • Stroke • Neurodegenerative disorders • Neuroimmunology
- Polysomnography • Sleep architecture

KEY POINTS

- Neurologic disorders impact the ability of the brain to generate sleep, wake, and circadian functions.
- Preexisting or de novo sleep-wake-circadian pathologies are generally underdiagnosed in neurologic patients despite their major impact on onset, evolution, and outcome of neurologic disorders.
- Neurologic disorders are frequently accompanied by sleep-wake EEG changes. Extensive brain damage can lead to the absence of measurable differentiation between sleep and wakefulness (status dissociatus).
- New technologies will facilitate early detection and (long-term) monitoring of neurologic patients and the optimization of their clinical management.

INTRODUCTION

The brain is the organ from which sleep, wakefulness, and circadian functions are generated and ultimately measured. The highly structured and timed transitions between wakefulness, non-rapid eye movement (NREM) sleep, and REM sleep requires an integration of neural networks across many brain structures, including the brainstem, subcortical regions such as the thalamus and hypothalamus, and basal forebrain.

Central nervous system (CNS) lesions underlying neurologic disorders can lead to primary sleep-wake and circadian disorders (SWCD) through lesioning of specific cell types or structures generating or regulating sleep, wake, and circadian functions or through nonspecific lesioning of diffuse neural networks. In addition, SWCD can arise secondarily from complications of CNS lesions such as spasticity, pain, and depression. In many cases SWCD may worsen over time, as in the case of progressive neurologic diseases.

[a] Department of Neurology, Bern University Hospital (Inselspital) and University Bern, Switzerland; [b] Ohio Sleep Medicine Institute, 4975 Bradenton Avenue, Dublin, OH 43017, USA; [c] Univ. Grenoble Alpes, Inserm, U1300, CHU Grenoble Alpes, Service Universitaire de Pneumologie Physiologie, Grenoble 38000, France; [d] Sensory-Motor System Lab, IRIS, ETH Zurich, Switzerland; [e] Department of Neurology, University of Sechenow, Moscow, Russia
[1] Present address: Schlaf-Wach-Epilepsie Zentrum (SWEZ), Universitätsklinik für Neurologie, Bern University Hospital, Inselspital, Freiburgstrasse 4, 3010 Bern, Switzerland.
* Corresponding author. Inselspital, Universitätsklinik für Neurologie CH-3010 Bern
E-mail address: markus.schmidt@insel.ch

Sleep Med Clin 16 (2021) 661–671
https://doi.org/10.1016/j.jsmc.2021.08.005
1556-407X/21/© 2021 The Author(s). Published by Elsevier Inc. This is an open access article under the CC BY-NC-ND license (http://creativecommons.org/licenses/by-nc-nd/4.0/).

Finally, SWCD may also represent the first or main manifestation of an underlying neurologic disorder such as dream enactment behavior in Parkinson disease (PD), excessive daytime sleepiness (EDS) in hypothalamic disorders, or insomnia in Alzheimer disease (AD).

Lesions of the various structures that regulate sleep, wake, and circadian functions will lead to specific changes. For example, lesions of the brainstem may affect aspects of REM sleep generation or expression, thalamic lesions can lead to a reduction of spindling, and damage to the suprachiasmatic nucleus may disrupt circadian rhythmicity. These various pathologic manifestations can be measured through subjective assessments, including questionnaires, and objective tools using actigraphy, polysomnography (PSG), or daytime vigilance testing (**Fig. 1**). The diversity of SWCD in neurologic patients, which may reflect brain damage or other factors such as comorbidities or medication, and their measurement in clinical practice are the subjects of this article.

STROKE

Stroke is one of the leading causes of death and disability worldwide[1] and is often associated with significant changes in sleep-wake electroencephalographic (EEG) architecture and circadian expression.[2,3] In addition, SWCD are also increasingly recognized as stroke risk factors and modulators of stroke outcome.[2,4,5] Therefore, SWCD diagnosis and management should be considered in stroke care pathways.

Subjective Assessments

The simplest way to assess subjective SWCD in patients with stroke is by using structured interview questions. A detailed sleep history addressing sleep habits before and following stroke, including estimated sleep needs (hours per day), can be easily gathered from patients or their relatives, even at hospital admission.[6,7] However, limited studies have assessed subjective sleep duration prestroke and poststroke and heralded conflicting results. A systematic study from our group conducted in 438 patients suggested an increased sleep duration following ischemic stroke with a gradual, but incomplete, return to baseline at 12 months.[8] An increase in sleep duration or need is particularly often found in patients with (bilateral) lesions of the paramedian thalamus.[6,9]

Symptoms such as fatigue, insomnia, and EDS are common after stroke.[10,11] Restless legs syndrome (RLS), in contrast, does not seem to be more prevalent after stroke than in the general population.[12] In a systematic study from our center over a follow-up period of 2 years, fatigue was found in up to 28%, insomnia in 28%, EDS in 14%, and RLS in 9% of patients with stroke (manuscript in preparation).

Sleep questionnaires such as the Epworth Sleepiness Scale, Fatigue Severity Scale, Insomnia

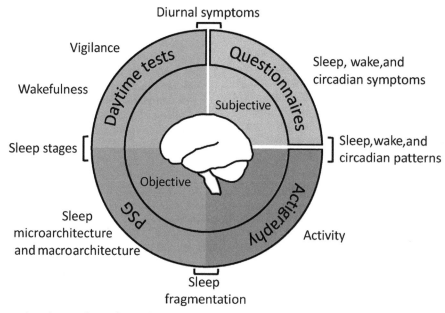

Fig. 1. Measuring sleep-wake and circadian disorders using subjective and objective assessments in neurologic disease.

Severity Index, and the Pittsburgh Sleep Quality Index Questionnaire[9,13,14] can also be used to help investigate specific symptoms of SWCD. It is important to note, however, that validation of these commonly used questionnaires as part of a test battery in patients with stroke is lacking. Moreover, the use of questionnaires for sleep-disordered breathing (SDB) has shown limitations in patients with stroke with their high sensitivity but a rather low specificity.[15] Taken together, although the use of questionnaires validated for the general population may provide potential screening tools for SWCD evaluation, objective assessments remain frequently necessary in a stroke population in which SWCD are highly prevalent.[16]

Objective Assessments

Circadian functions can be assessed using actigraphy. A disruption of circadian rhythmicity, as measured by core body temperature and actigraphy acutely after stroke, correlated strongly with functional outcome 3 months after stroke onset.[17] In addition to estimating macroparameters of sleep-wake rhythms, wearable devices may offer the possibility for long-term home monitoring, allowing the investigation of sleep-wake behavior evolution after stroke, as well as measuring the effect or efficacy of therapeutic interventions (see section 6.2).[18]

In-laboratory PSG demonstrates that sleep macroarchitectural changes following stroke potentially affect all sleep and EEG variables.[2,11] For example, supratentorial stroke may be followed by a reduction in REM sleep in a stroke severity-dependent manner and may persist for months.[19,20] Brainstem stroke lesions affecting the ventrolateral and tegmental areas in the pons can also reduce REM sleep or lead to REM sleep behavior disorder (see later), especially in the case of bilateral lesions.[21] Noteworthy, stroke in these regions may lead to a reduction in NREM sleep even in the absence of subjective sleep complaints.[21]

Thalamic strokes predominantly reduce sleep spindles and deeper NREM sleep stages.[6,9,22,23] Indeed, a reduction in sleep spindles after thalamic and supratentorial strokes[24,25] may occur as a function of lesion size.[19] Moreover, spindle power reduction in the peri-infarct area acutely after stroke is accompanied by a temporarily increased spindle power over the contralesional hemisphere.

In acute and chronic stroke, local slow-wave activity (SWA) is increased over the infarct area and decreased over the peri-infarct area during sleep[25]; this is of interest for different reasons. In a recent study we observed an association

between a reduction of the slow-wave slope in patients with thalamic stroke and daytime sleepiness.[26] In addition, SWA is increasingly linked with sleep-related learning and memory,[27,28] processes that could play a role in neuroplasticity after stroke.[5] In support of this hypothesis, optogenetically induced slow waves delivered during sleep were reported to improve functional outcomes in a mouse model of stroke.[29] Together, these data provide a conceptual framework for therapeutic noninvasive neuromodulation approaches targeting (slow wave) sleep after stroke (and overall brain injury).

Only a few studies objectively investigated the impact of stroke on daytime vigilance using the multiple sleep latency test (MSLT) and the maintenance of wakefulness test (MWT). Sleep latencies were reduced in subcortical stroke,[30] whereas the latencies did not necessarily correlate with subjective measures of EDS in patients with bilateral thalamic lesions.[22] These data reveal potential discrepancies between subjective questionnaires and objective monitoring that may reflect a discordance between perceived alertness and actual waking ability. Such discrepancies can also be observed in the general population[31] and reflect the need for objective assessments of daytime alertness. However, objective testing can be challenging because large supratentorial lesions may also limit the expression of EEG correlates of sleep-wake behaviors (see section Neurodegenerative Disorders).

NEURODEGENERATIVE DISORDERS

Sleep, wake, and circadian disturbances are a common finding in neurodegenerative diseases.[32] As neurodegenerative diseases often affect the neuronal networks underlying the generation of sleep, wakefulness, and circadian timing, standard methods to measure and score sleep and wakefulness are potentially challenging,[33] and this was dramatically documented by Landolt and colleagues[33] in study of patients with sleep-wake disturbances in the course of Creutzfeldt-Jakob disease. Similarly, Santamaria and colleagues[34] emphasized the importance of audiovideographic recordings, including calibration of measured variables with clearly awake periods with major sleep and wake bouts in patients with brain damage.[34]

Subjective Assessments

Up to 60% of patients with AD and 90% of patients with PD suffer from insomnia.[35,36] EDS is also frequent and may affect more than 40% to 50% of both patients with AD and those with PD.[36,37] REM sleep behavior disorder (RBD) is frequent in

PD[38] but rare in AD.[39] In RBD, the complex neural networks controlling muscle atonia or paralysis during REM sleep are disrupted, leading to motor activation during this stage of sleep. If RBD occurs in the context of a neurodegenerative disorder, such as PD, or is triggered by medication, it is classified as secondary RBD. However, if no underlying cause can be identified, it is known as idiopathic RBD (iRBD), which can appear in the prodromal phase of α-synucleinopathies. Finally, RLS is probably more prevalent in patients with PD compared with healthy individuals,[40] and, in patients with AD, RLS may manifest as nighttime agitation.[32]

Several questionnaires for RBD have been developed, including the RBD screening questionnaire (RBDSQ), which is the most commonly used.[38] A meta-analysis of the RBDSQ demonstrated a sensitivity and specificity of 91% and 77%, respectively.[41] However, this questionnaire demonstrated poor sensitivity and specificity in patients with PD.[41] Another problem common to all RBD questionnaires is that some patients are unable to complete the questionnaires, or they live alone and are unaware of their parasomnia. Finally, given the low prevalence of symptomatic RBD in the general population and assuming a questionnaire with a sensitivity and specificity of 90%, only approximately 10% of patients who screen positive will actually have RBD.[38] These and other data suggest the need for comprehensive objective assessments, particularly in patients with neurologic disorders.

Objective Assessments

Actigraphic measurements in patients with AD reveal alterations in sleep-wake patterns with irregular sleep-wake rhythms to a complete reversal of the day/night sleep pattern. Some of these changes can be observed in the prodromal phase of AD.[42] In PD, a loss of stability in the day-to-day rest-activity pattern is associated with impaired cognitive function,[43] whereas reduced circadian rhythmicity may be seen in the prodromal stage.[44] Finally, patients with iRBD show increased probable napping behavior, activity fragmentation, and physical inactivity during the active period. These rest-activity pattern alterations have been associated with an increased risk of phenoconversion to an overt α-synucleinopathy.[45]

Video-PSG assessments in patients with AD reveal reduced sleep efficiency and alterations in sleep macroarchitecture and microarchitecture (summarized in **Table 1**). As neurodegeneration progresses, electrographic features defining NREM stage 2 (N2) may disappear completely, rendering NREM stage 1 (N1) and N2 sleep practically indistinguishable. In this case, indeterminate NREM sleep may be scored.[34] This indeterminate NREM sleep may increase further with the disappearance of the slow waves in later stages of the disease.[46,47]

In patients with PD, the reduction in slow-wave sleep may be associated with increased periodic leg movements in sleep.[48] In addition, lower sigma power in NREM sleep may be predictive for cognitive impairment in PD.[50] In patients with iRBD, smaller densities of fast sleep spindles and larger densities of slow spindles are described.[51]

The diagnosis of an RBD requires the presence of muscle activity during REM sleep (REM sleep without atonia [RSWA]). RSWA shows some degree of night-to-night stability so that a single night of PSG is considered sufficient for the diagnosis of RBD.[38] Obstructive sleep apnea (OSA) is a common comorbidity in AD and PD. Importantly, patients with OSA may show motor events associated with respiratory effort in REM sleep,

Table 1		
Microarchitectural and macroarchitectural changes in Alzheimer and Parkinson disease		
	Alzheimer disease[46,47]	**Parkinson disease**[48,49]
Sleep efficiency	↓	↓
Slow wave sleep	↓	↓
REM sleep	↓ episode duration, with EEG slowing	↓
NREM sleep	N1 and N2 become indeterminate, later SW disappear	Lower sigma power
Microarchitecture	↓ frequency and amplitude of spindles and K-complexes	↓ frequency and amplitude of spindles
Sleep latency	↑	↑

Abbreviations: sigma, (12–15 Hz) reflects sleep spindle activity; SW, slow waves.

which can be misinterpreted as RBD, a finding referred to as pseudo-RBD.[52] If RBD is suspected in a patient with OSA, it is recommended to repeat the diagnostic workup after OSA treatment.[38]

When complex neuronal networks involved in the initiation and maintenance of sleep become increasingly impaired, components of different stages may occur together, leading to the so-called state dissociations. With increasing degeneration of these networks, state dissociations may increase in severity, culminating in a status dissociatus, characterized by a complete breakdown of state-determining boundaries.[53] Status dissociatus has been described in patients with α-synucleinopathies, as well as in other neurodegenerative and secondary brain diseases that predominantly affect the thalamus.[53]

Objective measurements using MSLT or MWT often reveal EDS in neurodegenerative disorders. Mean sleep latency was found to be significantly reduced in patients with AD when compared with healthy controls and to correlate with cognitive impairment.[54] Up to 50% of patients with PD suffer from EDS,[55] which is often underappreciated by patients.[37]

NEUROIMMUNOLOGICAL DISORDERS

Many neuroimmunological disorders affect CNS areas involved in regulating sleep, wakefulness, or circadian functions. In the case of narcolepsy type 1, a very specific group of neurons expressing hypocretin (orexin) in the hypothalamus is lost,[56,57] probably secondary to autoreactive CD4+ and CD8+ T cells.[58] Hypocretin neurons are essential for stabilizing the state of wakefulness, so their loss adversely affects the ability to maintain alertness.[57]

In contrast to a specific cell type affected in narcolepsy following a single inflammatory phase, multiple sclerosis (MS) is characterized by intermittent or chronic inflammatory-induced demyelination affecting different neuronal systems. Depending on the extent and localization of the lesions, a diverse range of symptoms can be observed, including SWCD. For example, MS lesions affecting the hypothalamus can result in secondary narcolepsy, whereas spinal lesions may trigger RLS or periodic limb movements in sleep.[59,60]

Subjective Assessments

The cardinal symptom in narcolepsy type 1 is cataplexy: sudden, short episodes with bilateral loss of muscle tone triggered by emotion. Although cataplexy is absent in narcolepsy type 2, all patients with narcolepsy complain of EDS[61] and may report disturbed sleep, episodes of sleep

paralysis, and hypnagogic (= while falling asleep) or hypnopompic (= while awakening) hallucinations.[56] Specific questionnaires for narcolepsy, such as the Swiss narcolepsy scale,[62] address this unique constellation of symptoms. In contrast, the Epworth sleepiness scale only assesses the symptom of EDS and shows high mean scores in patients with narcolepsy (17 ± 3 of 24).[61]

Fatigue in MS is found in greater than 85% of patients[63] and can be assessed by the Fatigue Severity Scale or by the Fatigue Scale for Motor and Cognitive Functions questionnaire developed for MS-related fatigue.[64] In contrast to fatigue, EDS is less consistent at the group level in MS, although it still may be present in a substantial subpopulation.[65] Pathologic fatigue and sleepiness in patients with MS was significantly associated with positive screenings for SDB, RLS, and insomnia in a large, questionnaire-based study.[66] Comorbid SDB is present in 12% to 80% of patients with MS, a prevalence likely exceeding that observed in the general population.[59,67] Finally, the prevalence of RLS was reported to be 4 times higher in patients with MS than in the general population.[59,68]

Patients with autoimmune encephalitis commonly suffer from sleep complaints such as insomnia, hypersomnolence, dream enactment behaviors, or frequent arousals.[69] The anti-IgLON5 syndrome is a rare autoimmune disease characterized by sleep-wake disturbances, including insomnia, excessive sleepiness, RBD, SDB, and neurologic manifestations such as bulbar dysfunction and gait and cognitive problems.[70]

Objective Assessments

Sleep-wake examinations involving PSG and MSLT assessments play a critical role for the diagnostic criteria of narcolepsy according to the International Classification of Sleep Disorders, third edition.[71] For example, the PSG may reveal a REM sleep latency within 15 minutes after sleep onset (sleep onset REM) in up to 50% of patients.[56] Furthermore, sleep fragmentation and reduced sleep efficiency are also characteristic for narcolepsy.[56] Current diagnostic criteria of narcolepsy rely on MSLT findings, which should document a mean sleep latency of 8 minutes or less and at least 2 naps with REM sleep.[71]

In patients with MS, PSG may reveal an increased arousal index and reduced sleep efficiency.[72] The MSLT can help to further evaluate sleepiness in patients with MS, for example, to exclude narcolepsy, but robust epidemiologic data on the MSLT in patients with MS are lacking.[59] In autoimmune encephalitis, PSG may show sleep fragmentation, reduced sleep efficiency, and reduced or absent NREM stage 3 (N3) and REM sleep.[69] In a small study, spindle density was shown to be decreased.[73] Larger systematic studies are needed to assess associations between antibody subtypes and specific sleep disorders and the influence of sleep disorders on the clinical presentation and long-term outcome of patients with autoimmune encephalitis. In the anti-IgLON5 syndrome, the PSG may show an abnormal (undifferentiated) NREM sleep initiation, with sleep-related vocalizations and movements, followed by periods of normal NREM sleep, RBD, and OSA with stridor.[74]

EPILEPSY

Epilepsy is linked in a bidirectional manner to sleep. On the one hand, seizures, antiepileptic drugs, and interictal activity may alter sleep macroarchitecture and microarchitecture. On the other hand, sleep deprivation and comorbid sleep disorders may reduce the seizure threshold and limit its control.[75] Moreover, up to one-half of epileptic patients report sleep complaints.[76,77] Specifically, 52% complain of sleep maintenance insomnia (vs 38% in controls), whereas loud snoring and restless legs symptoms were found to be independent predictors of EDS in patients with epilepsy.[76] Moderate to severe SDB affects up to 26.5% of epileptic patients and may increase seizure frequency.[78] These findings highlight the importance of SWCD diagnosis and treatment in epilepsy management. In addition, several epilepsy syndromes show seizure activity exclusively or predominantly in sleep. These are termed sleep-related epilepsy.

Subjective Measures

A careful clinical history with both patient and witness is critical to correctly diagnose and establish the semiology of the ictal events. The most frequent complaints are EDS and insomnia.[76,79] Specific questionnaires, such as the Frontal Lobe Epilepsy and Parasomnias scale, can help differentiate some forms of epilepsy from disorders of arousal (confusional arousal, sleepwalking and sleep terrors), although the semiological similarities pose diagnostic challenges.

Objective Measures

In case of suspicion of sleep-related epilepsy, objective measurements, such as home video recording and a video-PSG with extended EEG (10/20) montage is recommended.[80,81] PSG recordings in patients with epilepsy may show sleep architectural abnormalities, such as increased number of arousals and increased wake after sleep onset, increased stage shifts, and reduced percentage of REM sleep.[75] Epileptic activity is also specifically affected by sleep stage: interictal and ictal activity are increased predominantly in NREM sleep when compared with REM sleep.[82,83] This association is proposed to be associated with NREM sleep characteristics, that is, increased EEG synchronization that may favor seizure propagation and muscle tone preservation during NREM sleep that allows seizure-related movements to occur.[84]

Although sleepiness is a frequent complaint in patients with epilepsy, objective assessments of vigilance and wakefulness are sparse, showing little correlation between subjective and objective sleepiness.[85]

NEW FRONTIERS FOR MEASURING SLEEP-WAKE AND CIRCADIAN DISORDERS IN NEUROLOGIC DISORDERS

Given the high prevalence of sleep disorders comorbid with neurologic disorders and their impact on the course or presentation of neurologic disease, it is essential to identify and treat SWCD to optimize neurologic management. Future advancements are needed with respect to screening, including questionnaires specifically designed for patients with neurologic disorders. Moreover, future technologies on the horizon may promote new diagnostic and management tools.

Future Role of Questionnaires

Screening tools for individual SWCD disorders are available, including the Epworth Sleepiness Scale[86] to test the propensity to fall asleep, the Fatigue Severity Scale,[87] Insomnia Severity Index,[88] the Single Question for RLS,[89] STOP-BANG score for sleep apnea,[90] and the Swiss Narcolepsy Scale[62] to name a few. However, a fully validated general screening instrument for patients with neurologic disorders is currently missing, making it difficult for neurologists outside of sleep medicine to select the right screening tool. Therefore, a brief domain-based questionnaire might be the future such as a first promising attempt in the SDS-25.[91] The validation of a single, brief questionnaire covering a targeted spectrum of SWCD designed for patients with neurologic disorders remains an area of interest for future research.

Future Frontiers in Sleep-Wake and Circadian Disorders Monitoring

In-laboratory video PSG (ie, a level 1 sleep study) plays a central role in objective clinical sleep

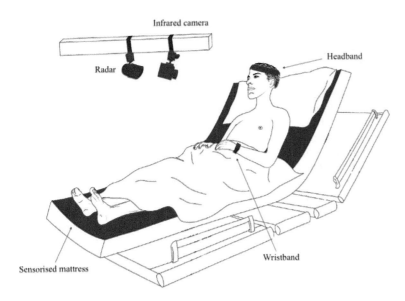

Fig. 2. Example of an unobtrusive sensor network. On top, 2 contactless technologies, radar and infrared camera. The subject lies on a sensorized mattress wearing a smart wristband and an electroencephalographic-based headband.[93]

Infrared camera

Headband

Radar

Wristband

Sensorised mattress

assessment. Although it is the current gold standard for diagnosis of many SWCD, the unnatural environment and highly obtrusive character of the currently used devices may negatively affect sleep. In addition, this single night snapshot cannot detect periodicities or subtle changes over time as may be anticipated for many chronic or progressive neurologic disorders.

With advances in technology, less obtrusive devices address these issues and allow long-term home monitoring of sleep, wake, and circadian functions. Actigraphy was one of the first wearable devices that could measure several parameters of the sleep-wake rhythm. Novel wrist bands have included additional sensors for measuring heart rate, skin temperature, and electrodermal activity.[92] To record brain activity and derive sleep stages, headbands with dry EEG electrodes have gained popularity over the last years.[93] Even less invasive are contactless technologies to monitor sleep. Here we find sensorized mattresses based on ballistocardiography, which are able to extract body movements, heart rate, and respiratory rate.[94] In addition, bedside radar technology has recently been suggested as a potential future tool for sleep-wake discrimination,[95] sleep stage scoring,[96] and detection of SDB.[97] Although skin temperature changes occur across sleep and wake states, the potential roles of other technologies such as thermal cameras or electrodermal activity remain unclear.

Several studies have shown a high correlation between such wearable and nearable devices and PSG.[98] However, studies mostly compared one single device to PSG in healthy participants. As a result, there is lack of ground truth data on

2 levels: first, each device records specific types of data, but it remains unclear what combination of sensing devices may be optimal. Second, studies are lacking to validate such devices as shown in **Fig. 2** in both medical and home settings with patients with sleep or neurologic disorders. The medical application of currently available commercial smartwatches has been complicated by the lack of harmonization of technologies across devices. However, if these and other wristband devices become validated in the future, the medical setting for clinic investigation will likely shift from an in-laboratory setting to the home environment. Theoretically, a combined sensor network offers the potential for long-term, in-home monitoring with a similar diagnostic efficacy as PSG. At our institution a new unit called Neuro-Tec was recently inaugurated to test and validate new approaches for wearable and nearable approaches to long-term and home monitoring of SWCD and other disturbances in neurologic patients.[99]

SUMMARY

Neurologic disorders often affect sleep-wake and circadian patterns, either as a primary consequence of brain lesions that disrupt neuronal networks regulating sleep or circadian time or as a secondary consequence of underlying sensory or motor neuropathology. These SWCD may present in diverse ways, ranging from changes to sleep structure or EEG microarchitecture without subjective symptoms up to the complete dissociation of the sleep-wake stages in advanced neurodegeneration. Identifying these symptoms using both subjective and objective assessments allows inference into the site of the lesion and progression of disease. Importantly, diagnosis and treatment of SWCD can optimize management of neurologic diseases.

The impact of neurologic disorders on SWCD is diverse as can be measured using various methods. Available tools not only provide objective assessments of nighttime sleep but also can provide a long-term view of circadian activity patterns through actigraphy or wearable devices. Moreover, objective daytime testing can measure diurnal symptoms that may result from SWCD. Finally, new technologies may potentially facilitate future long-term monitoring of chronic neurologic patients while retaining a high resolution of recording fidelity, thereby allowing optimization of clinical management and monitoring of treatment efficacy.

DISCLOSURE

S. Baillieul received support from the European Respiratory Society Fellowship through a Long-Term Research Fellowship (Fellowship ID number: LTRF202001-00711). C.L.A. Bassetti received support from the Swiss National Science Foundation grant titled Early Sleep Apnea Treatment in Stroke: A Randomized, Rater-Blinded, Clinical Trial of Adaptive Servo-Ventilation (Grant ID number: 33IC30_166827). M.H. Schmidt and C.L.A. Bassetti received support from the Interfaculty Research Cooperation (IRC): Decoding Sleep, University of Bern, Bern, Switzerland (Grant Identifier: 41-050). M.H. Schmidt received support from Innosuisse (Grant Identifier: 30664.1 IP-LS).

REFERENCES

1. Feigin VL, Vos T, Nichols E, et al. The global burden of neurological disorders: translating evidence into policy. Lancet Neurol 2020;19(3):255–65.
2. Gottlieb E, Landau E, Baxter H, et al. The bidirectional impact of sleep and circadian rhythm dysfunction in human ischaemic stroke: a systematic review. Sleep Med Rev 2019;45:54–69.
3. Hermann DM, Bassetti CL. Sleep-related breathing and sleep-wake disturbances in ischemic stroke. Neurology 2009;73(16):1313–22.
4. Bassetti CLA, Randerath W, Vignatelli L, et al. EAN/ERS/ESO/ESRS statement on the impact of sleep disorders on risk and outcome of stroke. Eur J Neurol 2020;27(7):1117–36.
5. Duss SB, Seiler A, Schmidt MH, et al. The role of sleep in recovery following ischemic stroke: a review of human and animal data. Neurobiol Sleep Circadian Rhythms 2017;2:94–105.
6. Hermann DM, Siccoli M, Brugger P, et al. Evolution of neurological, neuropsychological and sleep-wake disturbances after paramedian thalamic stroke. Stroke 2008;39(1):62–8.
7. Vock J, Achermann P, Bischof M, et al. Evolution of sleep and sleep EEG after hemispheric stroke. J Sleep Res 2002;11(4):331–8.
8. Dekkers M, Alexiev F, Denier N, et al. Sleep duration increases after stroke: a prospective study of 438 patients. Eur J Neurol 2020;27(suppl. 1):252.
9. Wu W, Cui L, Fu Y, et al. Sleep and cognitive abnormalities in acute minor thalamic infarction. Neurosci Bull 2016;32(4):341–8.
10. Maestri M, Romigi A, Schirru A, et al. Excessive daytime sleepiness and fatigue in neurological disorders. Sleep Breath 2020;24(2):413–24.
11. Bassetti CL. Sleep and stroke. In: Sleep medicine Textbook. 2nd Edition. European Sleep Research Society (ESRS); 2021. p. 959–70.
12. Hasan F, Gordon C, Wu D, et al. Dynamic prevalence of sleep disorders following stroke or transient ischemic Attack: systematic review and meta-analysis. Stroke 2021;52(2):655–63.
13. Chen X, Bi H, Zhang M, et al. Research of sleep disorders in patients with acute cerebral infarction. J Stroke Cerebrovasc Dis 2015;24(11):2508–13.
14. Boulos MI, Murray BJ, Muir RT, et al. Periodic limb movements and white matter Hyperintensities in first-Ever minor stroke or high-risk transient ischemic Attack. Sleep 2017;40(3). https://doi.org/10.1093/sleep/zsw080.
15. Takala M, Puustinen J, Rauhala E, et al. Pre-screening of sleep-disordered breathing after stroke: a systematic review. Brain Behav 2018;8(12):e01146.
16. Brown DL, He K, Kim S, et al. Prediction of sleep-disordered breathing after stroke. Sleep Med 2020;75:1–6.
17. Takekawa H, Miyamoto M, Miyamoto T, et al. Circadian rhythm abnormalities in the acute phase of cerebral infarction correlate with poor prognosis in the chronic phase. Auton Neurosci 2007;131(1–2):131–6.
18. Kwon S, Kim H, Yeo W-H. Recent advances in wearable sensors and portable electronics for sleep monitoring. iScience 2021;24(5):102461.
19. Bassetti CL, Aldrich MS. Sleep electroencephalogram changes in acute hemispheric stroke. Sleep Med 2001;2(3):185–94.
20. Pace M, Camilo MR, Seiler A, et al. Rapid eye movements sleep as a predictor of functional outcome after stroke: a translational study. Sleep 2018;41(10). https://doi.org/10.1093/sleep/zsy138.
21. Bassetti CL, Hermann DM. Sleep and stroke. Handbook Clin Neurol 2011;99:1051–72. https://doi.org/10.1016/B978-0-444-52007-4.00021-7. Elsevier.
22. Bassetti C, Mathis J, Gugger M, et al. Hypersomnia following paramedian thalamic stroke: a report of 12 patients. Ann Neurol 1996;39(4):471–80.

23. Mensen A, Poryazova R, Huber R, et al. Individual spindle detection and analysis in high-density recordings across the night and in thalamic stroke. Sci Rep 2018;8(1):17885.

24. Gottselig JM, Bassetti CL, Achermann P. Power and coherence of sleep spindle frequency activity following hemispheric stroke. Brain 2002;125(2): 373–83.

25. Poryazova R, Huber R, Khatami R, et al. Topographic sleep EEG changes in the acute and chronic stage of hemispheric stroke. J Sleep Res 2015;24(1):54–65.

26. Jaramillo V, Jendoubi J, Maric A, et al. Thalamic influence on slow wave slope renormalization during sleep. Ann Neurol 2021. https://doi.org/10.1002/ana.26217.

27. Diekelmann S, Born J. The memory function of sleep. Nat Rev Neurosci 2010;11(2):114–26. https://doi.org/10.1038/nrn2762.

28. Tononi G, Cirelli C. Sleep and the price of plasticity: from synaptic and cellular homeostasis to memory consolidation and integration. Neuron 2014;81(1): 12–34.

29. Facchin L, Schöne C, Mensen A, et al. Slow waves promote sleep-dependent plasticity and functional recovery after stroke. J Neurosci 2020;40(45): 8637–51.

30. Ding Q, Whittemore R, Redeker N. Excessive daytime sleepiness in stroke Survivors: an integrative review. Biol Res Nurs 2016;18(4):420–31.

31. Kim H, Young T. Subjective daytime sleepiness: Dimensions and correlates in the general population. Sleep 2005;28(5):625–34.

32. Peter-Derex L, Yammine P, Bastuji H, et al. Sleep and Alzheimer's disease. Sleep Med Rev 2015;19:29–38.

33. Landolt H-P, Glatzel M, Blattler T, et al. Sleep-wake disturbances in sporadic Creutzfeldt-Jakob disease. Neurology 2006;66(9):1418–24.

34. Santamaria J, Hogl B, Trenkwalder C, et al. Scoring sleep in neurologic patients: the need for specific considerations. Sleep 2011;34(10):1283–4.

35. Sani TP, Bond RL, Marshall CR, et al. Sleep symptoms in syndromes of frontotemporal dementia and Alzheimer's disease: a proof-of-principle behavioural study. eNeurologicalSci 2019;17:100212. https://doi.org/10.1016/j.ensci.2019.100212.

36. Rothman SM, Mattson MP. Sleep disturbances in Alzheimer's and Parkinson's diseases. Neuromol Med 2012;14(3):194–204.

37. Bargiotas P, Lachenmayer ML, Schreier DR, et al. Sleepiness and sleepiness perception in patients with Parkinson's disease: a clinical and electrophysiological study. Sleep 2019;42(4). https://doi.org/10.1093/sleep/zsz004.

38. Dauvilliers Y, Schenck CH, Postuma RB, et al. REM sleep behaviour disorder. Nat Rev Dis Primers 2018;4(1):19.

39. Galbiati A, Carli G, Hensley M, et al. REM sleep behavior disorder and Alzheimer's disease: Definitely No relationship? J Alzheimers Dis 2018;63(1):1–11.

40. Yang X, Liu B, Shen H, et al. Prevalence of restless legs syndrome in Parkinson's disease: a systematic review and meta-analysis of observational studies. Sleep Med 2018;43:40–6.

41. Li K, Li S-H, Su W, et al. Diagnostic accuracy of REM sleep behaviour disorder screening questionnaire: a meta-analysis. Neurol Sci 2017;38(6):1039–46.

42. Musiek ES, Bhimasani M, Zangrilli MA, et al. Circadian rest-activity pattern changes in aging and Preclinical Alzheimer disease. JAMA Neurol 2018;75(5):582.

43. Wu JQ, Li P, Stavitsky Gilbert K, et al. Circadian rest-activity rhythms Predict cognitive function in early Parkinson's disease independently of sleep. Mov Disord Clin Pract 2018;5(6):614–9.

44. Leng Y, Blackwell T, Cawthon PM, et al. Association of circadian abnormalities in Older Adults with an increased risk of developing Parkinson disease. JAMA Neurol 2020;77(10):1270.

45. Feng H, Chen L, Liu Y, et al. Rest-activity pattern alterations in idiopathic REM sleep behavior disorder. Ann Neurol 2020;88(4):817–29.

46. Petit D, Gagnon J-F, Fantini ML, et al. Sleep and quantitative EEG in neurodegenerative disorders. J Psychosom Res 2004;56(5):487–96.

47. McCurry SM, Ancoli-Israel S. Sleep dysfunction in Alzheimer's disease and other dementias. Curr Treat Options Neurol 2003;5(3):261–72.

48. Zhang F, Niu L, Liu X, et al. Rapid eye movement sleep behavior disorder and neurodegenerative diseases: an Update. Aging Dis 2020;11(2):315.

49. Christensen JAE, Nikolic M, Warby SC, et al. Sleep spindle alterations in patients with Parkinson's disease. Front Hum Neurosci 2015;9. https://doi.org/10.3389/fnhum.2015.00233.

50. Latreille V, Carrier J, Gaudet-Fex B, et al. Electroencephalographic prodromal markers of dementia across conscious states in Parkinson's disease. Brain 2016;139(4):1189–99.

51. O'Reilly C, Godin I, Montplaisir J, et al. REM sleep behaviour disorder is associated with lower fast and higher slow sleep spindle densities. J Sleep Res 2015;24(6):593–601.

52. Iranzo A, Santamaría J. Severe obstructive sleep apnea/Hypopnea Mimicking REM sleep behavior disorder. Sleep 2005;28(2):203–6.

53. Antelmi E, Ferri R, Iranzo A, et al. From state dissociation to status dissociatus. Sleep Med Rev 2016; 28:5–17.

54. Bonanni E, Maestri M, Tognoni G, et al. Daytime sleepiness in mild and moderate Alzheimer's disease and its relationship with cognitive impairment. J Sleep Res 2005;14(3):311–7.

55. Arnulf I. Excessive daytime sleepiness in parkinsonism. Sleep Med Rev 2005;9(3):185–200.

56. Bassetti CLA, Adamantidis A, Burdakov D, et al. Narcolepsy — clinical spectrum, aetiopathophysiology, diagnosis and treatment. Nat Rev Neurol 2019; 15(9):519–39.

57. Adamantidis AR, Schmidt MH, Carter ME, et al. A circuit perspective on narcolepsy. Sleep 2020; 43(5):zsz296.

58. Latorre D, Kallweit U, Armentani E, et al. T cells in patients with narcolepsy target self-antigens of hypocretin neurons. Nature 2018;562(7725):63–8.

59. Veauthier C. Sleep disorders in multiple sclerosis. Review. Curr Neurol Neurosci Rep 2015;15(5):21.

60. Kallweit U, Bassetti CLA, Oberholzer M, et al. Coexisting narcolepsy (with and without cataplexy) and multiple sclerosis: Six new cases and a literature review. J Neurol 2018;265(9):2071–8.

61. Luca G, Haba-Rubio J, Dauvilliers Y, et al. Clinical, polysomnographic and genome-wide association analyses of narcolepsy with cataplexy: a European Narcolepsy Network study. J Sleep Res 2013; 22(5):482–95.

62. Bargiotas P, Dietmann A, Haynes AG, et al. The Swiss Narcolepsy Scale (SNS) and its short form (sSNS) for the discrimination of narcolepsy in patients with hypersomnolence: a cohort study based on the Bern Sleep–Wake Database. J Neurol 2019; 266(9):2137–43.

63. Krupp LB, Alvarez LA, LaRocca NG, et al. Fatigue in multiple sclerosis. Arch Neurol 1988;45(4):435–7.

64. Penner I, Raselli C, Stöcklin M, et al. The Fatigue Scale for Motor and Cognitive Functions (FSMC): validation of a new instrument to assess multiple sclerosis-related fatigue. Mult Scler 2009;15(12): 1509–17.

65. Popp RFJ, Fierlbeck AK, Knüttel H, et al. Daytime sleepiness versus fatigue in patients with multiple sclerosis: a systematic review on the Epworth sleepiness scale as an assessment tool. Sleep Med Rev 2017;32:95–108.

66. Brass SD, Li C-S, Auerbach S. The Underdiagnosis of sleep disorders in patients with multiple sclerosis. J Clin Sleep Med 2014;10(09):1025–31.

67. Caminero A, Bartolomé M. Sleep disturbances in multiple sclerosis. J Neurol Sci 2011;309(1–2):86–91.

68. Italian REMS Study Group, Manconi M, Ferini-Strambi L, Filippi M, et al. Multicenter case-control study on restless legs syndrome in multiple sclerosis: the REMS study. Sleep 2008;31(7):944–52.

69. Blattner MS, Day GS. Sleep disturbances in patients with autoimmune encephalitis. Curr Neurol Neurosci Rep 2020;20(7):28.

70. Gaig C, Graus F, Compta Y, et al. Clinical manifestations of the anti-IgLON5 disease. Neurology 2017; 88(18):1736–43.

71. American Academy of Sleep Medicine, editor. International Classification of sleep disorders. 3. ed. American Acad. of Sleep Medicine; 2014.

72. Tanioka K, Castelnovo A, Tachibana N, et al. Framing multiple sclerosis under a polysomnographic perspective. Sleep. Published online October 22, 2019:zsz232. doi:10.1093/sleep/zsz232

73. Serdaroglu E, Tezer FI, Saygi S. Autoimmune epilepsy and/or limbic encephalitis can lead to changes in sleep spindles. Noro Psikiyatr Ars 2017;8. https://doi.org/10.5152/npa.2017.19442. Published online September.

74. Gaig C, Iranzo A, Santamaria J, et al. The sleep disorder in anti-IgLON5 disease. Curr Neurol Neurosci Rep 2018;18(7):41.

75. Kataria L, Vaughn BV. Sleep and epilepsy. Sleep Med Clin 2016;11(1):25–38.

76. Khatami R, Zutter D, Siegel A, et al. Sleep-wake habits and disorders in a series of 100 adult epilepsy patients—a prospective study. Seizure 2006; 15(5):299–306.

77. Matsuoka E, Saji M, Kanemoto K. Daytime sleepiness in epilepsy patients with special attention to traffic accidents. Seizure 2019;69:279–82.

78. Sivathamboo S, Perucca P, Velakoulis D, et al. Sleep-disordered breathing in epilepsy: epidemiology, mechanisms, and treatment. Sleep 2018; 41(4). https://doi.org/10.1093/sleep/zsy015.

79. Quigg M, Gharai S, Ruland J, et al. Insomnia in epilepsy is associated with continuing seizures and worse quality of life. Epilepsy Res 2016;122:91–6. https://doi.org/10.1016/j.eplepsyres.2016.02.014.

80. Nobili L, Weerd A, Rubboli G, et al. Standard procedures for the diagnostic pathway of sleep-related epilepsies and comorbid sleep disorders: an EAN, ESRS and ILAE-Europe consensus review. Eur J Neurol 2021;28(1):15–32.

81. Wu T, Avidan AY, Engel J. Sleep and epilepsy, clinical spectrum and Updated review. Sleep Med Clin 2021;16(2):389–408.

82. Frauscher B, von Ellenrieder N, Ferrari-Marinho T, et al. Facilitation of epileptic activity during sleep is mediated by high amplitude slow waves. Brain 2015;138(Pt 6):1629–41.

83. Zubler F, Rubino A, Lo Russo G, et al. Correlating interictal Spikes with sigma and Delta Dynamics during non-rapid-eye-movement-sleep. Front Neurol 2017;8:288. https://doi.org/10.3389/fneur.2017.00288.

84. Shouse MN, Farber PR, Staba RJ. Physiological basis: how NREM sleep components can promote and REM sleep components can suppress seizure discharge propagation. Clin Neurophysiol 2000;111:S9–18. https://doi.org/10.1016/S1388-2457(00)00397-7.

85. Drake ME, Weate SJ, Newell SA, et al. Multiple sleep latency tests in epilepsy. Clin Electroencephalogr 1994;25(2):59–62.

86. Johns MW. A new method for measuring daytime sleepiness: the Epworth sleepiness scale. Sleep 1991;14(6):540–5.

87. Krupp LB. The fatigue severity scale: application to patients with multiple sclerosis and systemic Lupus Erythematosus. Arch Neurol 1989;46(10):1121.

88. Gagnon C, Belanger L, Ivers H, et al. Validation of the insomnia severity index in primary care. J Am Board Fam Med 2013;26(6):701–10.

89. Ferri R, Lanuzza B, Cosentino FII, et al. A single question for the rapid screening of restless legs syndrome in the neurological clinical practice. Eur J Neurol 2007;14(9):1016–21.

90. Chung F, Subramanyam R, Liao P, et al. High STOP-Bang score indicates a high probability of obstructive sleep apnoea. Br J Anaesth 2012;108(5):768–75.

91. Klingman JK, Jungquist CR, Perlis ML. Introducing the sleep disorders symptom Checklist-25: a primary care Friendly and comprehensive screener for sleep disorders. Sleep Med Res 2017;8(1):17–25.

92. De Zambotti M, Cellini N, Goldstone A, et al. Wearable sleep technology in clinical and research settings. Med Sci Sports Exerc 2019;51(7):1538–57.

93. Arnal PJ, Thorey V, Debellemaniere E, et al. Original Article the Dreem Headband compared to polysomnography for electroencephalographic signal acquisition and sleep staging. Sleep 2020;1–13. https://doi.org/10.1093/sleep/zsaa097.

94. Xie Q, Wang M, Zhao Y, et al. A Personalized Beat-to-Beat heart rate detection system from Ballistocardiogram for smart home applications. IEEE Trans Biomed Circuits Syst 2019;13(6):1593–602.

95. Heglum HSA, Kallestad H, Vethe D, et al. Distinguishing sleep from wake with a radar sensor: a contact-free real-time sleep monitor. Sleep 2021;44(8). https://doi.org/10.1093/sleep/zsab060. zsab060.

96. Toften S, Pallesen S, Hrozanova M, et al. Validation of sleep stage classification using non-contact radar technology and machine learning (Somnofy®). Sleep Med 2020;75:54–61. https://doi.org/10.1016/j.sleep.2020.02.022.

97. Zhou Y, Shu D, Xu H, et al. Validation of novel automatic ultra-wideband radar for sleep apnea detection. J Thorac Dis 2020;12(4):1286–95.

98. Mantua J, Gravel N, Spencer RMC. Reliability of sleep measures from four personal health monitoring devices compared to research-based actigraphy and polysomnography. Sensors (Switzerland) 2016;16(5). https://doi.org/10.3390/s16050646.

99. Schindler KA, Nef T, Baud MO, et al. NeuroTec Sitem-Insel bern: Closing the last mile in Neurology. CTN 2021;5(2):13.

UNITED STATES POSTAL SERVICE ® Statement of Ownership, Management, and Circulation (All Periodicals Publications Except Requester Publications)

1. Publication Title	2. Publication Number	3. Filing Date
SLEEP MEDICINE CLINICS	025 – 053	9/18/2021

4. Issue Frequency	5. Number of Issues Published Annually	6. Annual Subscription Price
MAR, JUN, SEP, DEC	4	$225.00

7. Complete Mailing Address of Known Office of Publication (Not printer) (Street, city, county, state, and ZIP+4®)

ELSEVIER INC.
230 Park Avenue, Suite 800
New York, NY 10169

Contact Person
Malathi Samayan

Telephone (Include area code)
91-44-4299-4507

8. Complete Mailing Address of Headquarters or General Business Office of Publisher (Not printer)

ELSEVIER INC.
230 Park Avenue, Suite 800
New York, NY 10169

9. Full Names and Complete Mailing Addresses of Publisher, Editor, and Managing Editor (Do not leave blank)

Publisher (Name and complete mailing address)

Editor (Name and complete mailing address)

Joanna Collett, ELSEVIER INC.
1600 JOHN F KENNEDY BLVD. SUITE 1800
PHILADELPHIA, PA 19103-2899

Managing Editor (Name and complete mailing address)

Patrick Manley, ELSEVIER INC.
1600 JOHN F KENNEDY BLVD. SUITE 1800
PHILADELPHIA, PA 19103-2899

10. Owner (Do not leave blank. If the publication is owned by a corporation, give the name and address of the corporation immediately followed by the names and addresses of all stockholders owning or holding 1 percent or more of the total amount of stock. If not owned by a corporation, give the names and addresses of the individual owners. If owned by a partnership or other unincorporated firm, give its name and address as well as those of each individual owner. If the publication is published by a nonprofit organization, give its name and address.)

Full Name	Complete Mailing Address
WHOLLY OWNED SUBSIDIARY OF REED/ELSEVIER, US HOLDINGS	1600 JOHN F KENNEDY BLVD. SUITE 1800 PHILADELPHIA, PA 19103-2899

11. Known Bondholders, Mortgagees, and Other Security Holders Owning or Holding 1 Percent or More of Total Amount of Bonds, Mortgages, or Other Securities. If none, check box ▶ ☐ None

Full Name	Complete Mailing Address
N/A	

12. Tax Status (For completion by nonprofit organizations authorized to mail at nonprofit rates) (Check one)
The purpose, function, and nonprofit status of this organization and the exempt status for federal income tax purposes:
☒ Has Not Changed During Preceding 12 Months
☐ Has Changed During Preceding 12 Months (Publisher must submit explanation of change with this statement)

PS Form **3526**, July 2014 [Page 1 of 4 (see instructions page 4)] PSN: 7530-01-000-9931   PRIVACY NOTICE: See our privacy policy on www.usps.com.

13. Publication Title		14. Issue Date for Circulation Data Below
SLEEP MEDICINE CLINICS		JUNE 2021

15. Extent and Nature of Circulation			Average No. Copies Each Issue During Preceding 12 Months	No. Copies of Single Issue Published Nearest to Filing Date
a. Total Number of Copies (Net press run)			240	192
b. Paid Circulation (By Mail and Outside the Mail)	(1)	Mailed Outside-County Paid Subscriptions Stated on PS Form 3541 (Include paid distribution above nominal rate, advertiser's proof copies, and exchange copies)	170	139
	(2)	Mailed In-County Paid Subscriptions Stated on PS Form 3541 (Include paid distribution above nominal rate, advertiser's proof copies, and exchange copies)	0	0
	(3)	Paid Distribution Outside the Mails Including Sales Through Dealers and Carriers, Street Vendors, Counter Sales, and Other Paid Distribution Outside USPS®	36	29
	(4)	Paid Distribution by Other Classes of Mail Through the USPS (e.g., First-Class Mail®)	0	0
c. Total Paid Distribution (Sum of 15b (1), (2), (3), and (4))		▶	206	168
d. Free or Nominal Rate Distribution (By Mail and Outside the Mail)	(1)	Free or Nominal Rate Outside-County Copies Included on PS Form 3541	23	14
	(2)	Free or Nominal Rate In-County Copies Included on PS Form 3541	0	0
	(3)	Free or Nominal Rate Copies Mailed at Other Classes Through the USPS (e.g., First-Class Mail)	0	0
	(4)	Free or Nominal Rate Distribution Outside the Mail (Carriers or other means)	0	0
e. Total Free or Nominal Rate Distribution (Sum of 15d (1), (2), (3) and (4))		▶	23	14
f. Total Distribution (Sum of 15c and 15e)		▶	229	182
g. Copies not Distributed (See instructions to Publishers #4 (page #3))		▶	11	10
h. Total (Sum of 15f and g)		▶	240	192
i. Percent Paid (15c divided by 15f times 100)			89.95%	92.30%

If you are claiming electronic copies, go to line 16 on page 3. If you are not claiming electronic copies, skip to line 17 on page 3.

16. Electronic Copy Circulation		Average No. Copies Each Issue During Preceding 12 Months	No. Copies of Single Issue Published Nearest to Filing Date
a. Paid Electronic Copies	▶		
b. Total Paid Print Copies (Line 15c) + Paid Electronic Copies (Line 16a)	▶		
c. Total Print Distribution (Line 15f) + Paid Electronic Copies (Line 16a)	▶		
d. Percent Paid (Both Print & Electronic Copies) (16b divided by 16c × 100)	▶		

☒ I certify that 50% of all my distributed copies (electronic and print) are paid above a nominal price.

17. Publication of Statement of Ownership

☒ If the publication is a general publication, publication of this statement is required. Will be printed ☐ Publication not required.
in the DECEMBER 2021 issue of this publication.

18. Signature and Title of Editor, Publisher, Business Manager, or Owner

Malathi Samayan

Malathi Samayan - Distribution Controller

Date 9/18/2021

I certify that all information furnished on this form is true and complete. I understand that anyone who furnishes false or misleading information on this form or who omits material or information requested on the form may be subject to criminal sanctions (including fines and imprisonment) and/or civil sanctions (including civil penalties).

PS Form **3526**, July 2014 (Page 3 of 4)   PRIVACY NOTICE: See our privacy policy on www.usps.com